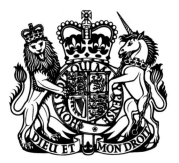

Independence, Well-being and Choice

Our vision for the future of social care for adults in England

Presented to Parliament
by the Secretary of State for Health
by Command of Her Majesty

March 2005

Cm 6499

£19.25

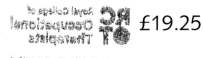

Contents

Preface

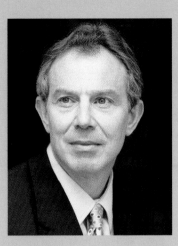

Independence, Well-being and Choice sets out our vision for the future of adult social care in England. The Green Paper addresses the challenges for social care of a changing and ageing population, higher expectations, and our desire to retain control over our own lives for as long as possible and over as much as possible.

It is family and friends, of course, who still take on most of the caring responsibilities. This support is given willingly but must not be taken for granted. Carers need not just society's thanks but also our support. But the realities of modern life mean that families are likely to be far more geographically scattered than in the past. Family breakdowns can also lead to less support being readily available while the great advances in healthcare mean we are all likely to live much longer with greater pressures on carers who themselves are becoming older. For these reasons alone, the daily, unfaltering support of thousands of dedicated workers in the formal social care system is likely to become more important in future years.

But we must continue adapting this support to ensure it meets people's expectations of a high-quality service and their aspirations for independence. This is an important part of our commitment to renew and modernise all our public services so they are centred on the needs and wishes of the individual. It is a tough challenge. But we have already seen in social care how the use of direct payments, for example, has helped improve services and transform lives.

Our task now is to continue this transformation right across the field of social care for adults so people are given more choice, higher quality support and greater control over their lives. We need to ensure the services we deliver are flexible and responsive enough to meet the differing needs and wishes of individuals. We must build on what works and learn from the experience and knowledge of front-line staff. And we must continue investing in the workforce so they have the training and skills to deliver the services people want and deserve.

The support we give to each other is one of the hallmarks of a decent society. I am certain that *Independence, Well-being and Choice* is the first step in making the transformation of social care a reality and I look forward to the debate that our proposals will stimulate.

Tony Blair

Rt Hon Tony Blair MP
The Prime Minister

Foreword

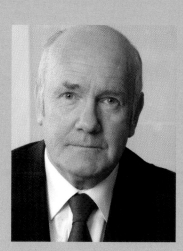

We live in a society in which people and organisations work together to provide support to those among us who need that support. The underpinning belief that every individual can expect support and care in times of need is a fundamental value of any good society. And most of this care and support we give freely to one another is part of basic relationships between us as social, caring people. As much as we can be, we are here for our children, family, friends and neighbours when they need us and we hope that they will support us in turn when we need them. The strength of our society and community is that it is built upon these practical expressions of the love and concern which form part of our close reciprocal relationships.

At another, more altruistic level, we sometimes care for strangers when their need is apparent and we have the time and ability to respond. These attitudes and behaviours are the important bedrock of our society and are more common than some may think.

But such care is not always enough.

In our modern society where people can become isolated, where extended families move around the country, work means that people are away from home and our lives seem to separate us from our neighbours, there are times when family and friends are not around to help.

There are also times when the needs of individuals are beyond what is possible for a family to manage without additional support. And, of course, people do not always want to be entirely dependent on friends and family. It is in these situations that organised social care should provide the services needed to ensure well-being and support the independence of individuals. We need social care to be organised to provide the right support to us when we need it.

This matters to us all. Social services and social care for adults touch all our lives at some time or another and, because of that, they are not about 'other' people. They are about families and friends, neighbours and communities, in the towns and in the countryside in every corner of England.

Organised social care supports the care we give each other. For many of us we need it to work together with our own informal care arrangements. And we will often seek specialist advice and support from voluntary and community organisations.

This is true in many varied circumstances: the couple filled with doubts and fears about the future when they learn that one of them has the early signs of dementia, someone who until now has enjoyed good health and a successful career; the young man who after years of drug and alcohol misuse and a string of prison sentences is trying to make sense of his life through seeking qualifications and a job; the woman with learning disabilities wondering how to support her parents, who care for her, and juggling those worries with her own concern about how she will manage in the future; an older woman with sight and hearing loss, living alone and becoming increasingly confused and easy prey to financial abuse from casual callers and junk mail.

Independence, Well-being and Choice is primarily about improving the organisation of social care by the voluntary and community sector and by government agencies to ensure it better serves the needs of those it supports. We want to give individuals and their friends and families greater control over the way in which social care supports their needs. We want to support carers to care and individuals to live as independently as possible for as long as possible.

We need to ensure modern care services are flexible enough to deliver support arrangements in partnership with others. Because we forget the bedrock of care, carried out by family, friends and neighbours at our peril. The nation depends upon the emotions and care that we all give to the people we know. If this relationship were to disappear, organised social care could not cope. We must never forget that.

Organised social care only works because of the support that the social care workforce provides to tens of thousands of people every day. These people combine the vital gift of caring with their work. Without that, social care in our society would collapse.

While as a nation we are proud of the people who provide social care, *Independence, Well-being and Choice* argues for change. It recognises that

sometimes the design and delivery of services are less effective than all of us would like them to be.

Sometimes:

- we involve social care staff at the wrong time;
- we ask people to adapt to the services we can offer, rather than adapting services to better meet their needs;
- too often the services we provide reduce, rather than increase, the control people have over their own lives; and
- most importantly they too often fail to treat adults who need social care as adults, often generating dependence rather than independence.

So sometimes social care is not provided as it should be.

And the demand for social care is growing. Every day that goes by our population is getting older, and more people are needing support. More children with complex and multiple disabilities are surviving into adulthood, and the number of people with mental health problems is increasing. We need new and better ways of providing support. Ways that reflect the world we live in today, not ones that are rooted in the past.

Our society, quite rightly, values the independence that we all try to develop as adults: our own income, our own family and our own choices for leisure, meals and lifestyle. That is why, in future, social care should be about helping people maintain their independence, leaving them with control over their lives, and giving them real choice over those lives, including the services they use. Services must recognise the changing world, our changing attitudes and our ageing population.

That is why we announced last April that we would develop a new 'vision' for adult social care. Since then we have consulted a range of stakeholders and used their feedback to produce *Independence, Well-being and Choice*.

Our vision is one where the social inclusion of adults with needs for care or support is promoted by:

- ensuring that, wherever possible, adults are treated as adults and that the provision of social care is not based upon the idea that a person's need for that care reduces them to total dependency;
- ensuring that people using services, their families and carers are put at the centre of assessing their own needs and given real choice about how those needs are met;
- improving access, not only to social care services, but to the full range of universal public services;
- shifting the focus of delivery to a more proactive, preventative model of care;
- recognising that carers also need support and that their well-being is central to the delivery of high-quality care; and
- empowering the social care workforce to be more innovative and to take the risk of enabling people to make their own life choices, where it is appropriate to do so.

Some of the ideas in this paper are new and build on examples of good practice from up and down the country. There are innovative 'pilot projects' where we can catch a glimpse of the future and many of these have informed our vision.

Although *Independence, Well-being and Choice* is the result of widespread consultation, it is itself a consultation document. We now look forward to hearing your views.

Dr John Reid MP
Secretary of State for Health

Executive summary

INTRODUCTION

Independence, Well-being and Choice is a consultation paper setting out proposals for the future direction of social care for all adults of all age groups in England.[1] Following the announcement in April 2004 that we would develop a new 'vision' for adult social care, we have consulted a number of stakeholders from inside and outside government, including people who use social care services. Those discussions have helped us to develop this paper and to ensure that our proposals are based on what people, both public and professional, have told us they would like to see in the future. Nevertheless, the policies and proposals contained within this paper are not fixed and we now welcome your views on the framework set out in this consultation.[2]

OUR VISION FOR ADULT SOCIAL CARE

Our starting point is the principle that everyone in society has a positive contribution to make to that society and that they should have a right to control their own lives. Our vision is to ensure that these values will drive the way we provide social care.

The vision we have for social care is one where:

- services help maintain the independence of the individual by giving them greater choice and control over the way in which their needs are met;
- the local authority and Director of Adult Social Services (DASS) have key strategic and leadership roles and work with a range of partners, including primary care trusts (PCTs) and the independent and voluntary sectors, to provide services which are well planned and integrated, make the most effective use of available resources, and meet the needs of a diverse community;
- local authorities give high priority to the inclusion of all sections of the community, and other agencies, including the NHS, recognise their own contribution to this agenda;
- services are of high quality and delivered by a well-trained workforce or by informal and family carers who are themselves supported;
- we make better use of technology to support people, and provide a wide range of supported housing options;
- we provide services with an emphasis on preventing problems and ensure that social care and the NHS work on a shared agenda to help maintain the independence of individuals;

- people with the highest needs receive the support and protection needed to ensure their own well-being and the safety of society; and
- the risks of independence for individuals are shared with them and balanced openly against benefits.

We have set out an ambitious programme for the next 10 to 15 years of services which will be person-centred, proactive and seamless. The lives of people who use social care will be transformed by giving them more control and choice.

WHY DO WE NEED A NEW VISION?

The Government's programme of reform of public services provides us with an opportunity to create a framework for social care which meets the requirements of the 21st century. Changes in population and communities mean that we are living longer but are less likely to be part of a close-knit family providing support. Communities are more diverse and existing services do not always recognise that. Society has higher expectations and people want greater control over their own lives, including the management of risk. In future, there will be competing demands on the workforce available.

It is therefore not realistic to plan to continue to deliver care in the way we have in the past. These challenges – the increased public expectation that people should be able to live with their own risk; increased geographical mobility, leading to the diminution of the support of the extended family; and the increased demand for organised social care – can only be met by reassessing the way in which social care is delivered.

SETTING CLEAR OUTCOMES

Care, and the support it provides, is one of the core values of our society. Where support from family and friends is not enough, it is supplemented by more formal models offered by the statutory, independent, voluntary and community sectors. We propose clear outcomes

for social care, derived from what people have told us they want, including:

- improved health;
- improved quality of life;
- making a positive contribution;
- exercise of choice and control;
- freedom from discrimination or harassment;
- economic well-being; and
- personal dignity.

These outcomes will be used to test and challenge how far social care is moving towards delivering the vision.

PUTTING PEOPLE IN CONTROL: IMPROVING ASSESSMENT, DIRECT PAYMENTS AND INDIVIDUAL BUDGETS

We want to move to a system where adults are able to take greater control of their lives. We want to encourage a debate about risk management and the right balance between protecting individuals and enabling them to manage their own risks. We want to provide better information and signposting to allow people to retain responsibility, and to put people at the centre of assessing their own needs and how those needs can best be met.

For too long social work has been perceived as a gatekeeper or rationer of services and has been accused, sometimes unfairly, of fostering dependence rather than independence. We want to create a different environment, which reinforces the core social work values of supporting individuals to take control of their own lives, and to make the choices which matter to them. We therefore emphasise the role that skilled social work will continue to play in assessing the needs of people with complex problems and in developing constructive relationships with people who need long-term support.

The greater appetite for people to retain more responsibility for their own life may at times conflict with the view of wider society and the media about the need to adopt a more protective stance. We would welcome a more open debate about risk management and what it means, which would enable social care staff to operate within a more supportive framework while meeting the legitimate aspirations of the people who use their services.

As part of our ambition to involve people much more closely in deciding how their needs should be met, we seek views on giving individuals the 'right to request' not to live in a residential setting.

We examine whether the single assessment process (SAP), the care programme approach (CPA) and person-centred planning (PCP) could be developed to provide an assessment tool for use with all people with complex needs.

We explore the possibility of streamlining assessments between agencies, particularly between local authorities and the Department for Work and Pensions.

We want to give people greater choice and control over how their needs should be met. In talking to people who use services and to carers, it is clear that direct payments[3] give people that choice and control, and we think that this is a mechanism that should be extended and encouraged where possible.

We would therefore like to encourage more people to consider whether direct payments are right for them, particularly in groups where take-up has been low, such as older people, people with mental health problems and young people moving to adult services.

We also want to consider ways of extending the benefits of direct payments to those currently excluded, by using an agent for those without the capacity to consent or unable to manage, even with assistance.

We think that all groups have the potential to benefit from the opportunity to have greater control over the services they need and how these should be provided, in a way that offers the real benefits of choice and control of direct

payments without the potential burdens. Therefore, building on the model of the In Control pilots for people with learning disabilities, and on the recommendations of the Prime Minister's Strategy Unit report *Improving the Life Chances of Disabled People,*[4] we propose to test the introduction of 'individual budgets' for adults with a disability or with an assessed need for social care support.

We will also consider whether a range of other budgets, for example community care resources and social services expenditure on minor equipment and adaptations, Independent Living Funds, the Family Fund and Access to Work, should also be included and test this, where appropriate, through pilots.

THE ROLE OF THE WIDER COMMUNITY

We emphasise the importance of carers and the need to ensure they are integral to the vision.

We also want to encourage a more flexible approach to putting together care packages using the wider resources of the community. This could include a mixture of more traditional social care services, use of universal services already provided by the local authority, and a contribution from the local voluntary and community sector (VCS).

In future, greater focus should be placed on preventative services through the wider well-being agenda and through better targeted, early interventions that prevent or defer the need for more costly intensive support. Current eligibility criteria allow for early intervention and support. More use of universal services could help people remain better integrated in their communities, prevent social isolation and maintain independence. This will allow social care to play its specialist and essential role in supporting those with specific needs that cannot be met in this way.

FUNDING

We set out the scale of social care spending, which runs at £14.4 billion of public funds in 2004/05, and identify scope for making better use of funding.

The changes proposed in *Independence, Well-being and Choice* will need to be met from existing funds. That is why we have suggested that this is a vision for the next 10 to 15 years. We know that change of this order cannot be introduced overnight and that local organisations will need time to manage the transition required for the introduction of individual budgets and greater choice for those who need support.

This raises some questions about how the proposals fit with *Fair Access to Care Services* (FACS) and how eligibility criteria can be set up to encompass both higher levels of need and early intervention.

We do expect that overall the proposals in this Green Paper will be cost-neutral for local authorities. However, in developing any detailed proposals as a result of this consultation the Department of Health (DH) will look closely at the cost implications for individual local authorities, taking account of our commitment to the New Burdens Doctrine.

CREATING THE RIGHT ENVIRONMENT

If our vision for social care is to be achieved, we need to look again at how we create the right environment in which the values and outcomes can be embedded and implemented.

The second part of the paper is dedicated to looking at:

- the strategic and leadership role that must be played by local government;
- strengthening joint working between health and social care services to deliver our vision;
- service improvement and delivery;
- the modernising of regulation and performance assessment;
- challenges facing the workforce; and
- building and supporting the VCS to extend the range and quality of services.

THE STRATEGIC AND LEADERSHIP ROLE OF LOCAL GOVERNMENT

We underline the vital leadership role played by local government, in particular by the Director of Adult Social Services (DASS). We are also publishing best practice guidance for consultation simultaneously on the role of the DASS and would welcome views on this separately.

We have recommended that the DASS and local authority should undertake regular needs assessments which look forward over the next 10 to 15 years and take account of the care needs of the whole population. These needs assessments will underline the role of local authorities in stimulating the local care service market to ensure the maximum range of choice for people who use services regardless of whether they pay for the services themselves or whether they are funded through social services budgets.

STRATEGIC COMMISSIONING

We assert the need to develop a strategic commissioning framework across all partners, to ensure the right balance between prevention, meeting low-level needs and providing intensive care and support for those with high-level complex needs.

To achieve the vision and its outcomes, local partners will need to work together to promote and ensure a strategic balance of investment in local services for:

- the general population, aimed at promoting health and social inclusion;
- people with emerging needs, to provide support to enable them to maintain their independence; and
- those with high-level complex needs, to provide intensive care and support.

Local partners will need to recognise the diversity of their local population and ensure that there is a range of services, which meet the needs of all members of the local community.

We also explore mechanisms for strengthening collaborative and partnership working.

Experience shows that where there is a will to work jointly there is an ability to overcome barriers to improve outcomes. Where the will does not exist, formal structures are not enough. We do not want to impose solutions. Decisions about the best models to suit local circumstances should be made locally. **However, we are clear that doing nothing will not be an option**. We expect the local health and social care communities to work together with other voluntary and statutory agencies to take a community-wide approach to commissioning.

SERVICE IMPROVEMENT AND DELIVERY

Alongside the challenge to improve the strategic commissioning of services is the task of improving their design and delivery. This will mean radically different ways of working, redesign of job roles and reconfiguration of services. This will call for skills in leadership, communications and management of change of the highest order.

We recognise the challenges faced in improving the design and delivery of services. We accept that better services and improved outcomes should be built on a firm knowledge base. We also accept that local providers need support to consider how services can be redesigned and refocused to provide the outcomes we have identified. We have created a Care Service Improvement Partnership to provide that support and are keen to ensure that existing good practice is spread right across the system.

We have also identified a number of examples of innovative practice, many of which are already in existence up and down the country, to illustrate that changes to traditional patterns of service can be achieved for the benefit of people using services. We hope that these examples will stimulate a wider debate.

REGULATION AND PERFORMANCE MANAGEMENT

We have highlighted the importance of regulation and performance management as levers for challenge and change and propose that both should be modernised to reflect more accurately the outcomes we have defined.

As services become more people-focused and more integrated across social care and health boundaries, existing inspection and performance management frameworks will play an important part in ensuring that our proposed outcomes and the vision are being delivered. The time is now right to modernise the approach to social care regulation, to be more proportionate, to reflect the aspirations of people using services properly, and to capture the quality and outcomes of the services provided. We have agreed with the Commission for Social Care Inspection (CSCI) that it should take forward a programme of work to formulate proposals for modernising regulation. In parallel, we will be reviewing the relevant national minimum standards and associated regulations.

We have now agreed in principle to merge CSCI and the Healthcare Commission into a single body by 2008, reflecting the increasing joint work between adult social care and health. The planned merger reflects shared objectives for the highest possible standards for everyone using social care and health services.

In summary, we plan to work to support delivery of our objectives through:

- aligning headline targets across relevant services with the objectives and outcomes we want;
- working with the inspectorates, local government and other stakeholders to develop performance measures and indicators that reflect and underpin the objectives, promote continuous improvement; and

- ensure that regulation, performance assessment and management systems for social care, the NHS and other services, promote these objectives and local joint working towards them.

THE WORKFORCE

People who use social care services say that the service is only as good as the person delivering it. They value social care practitioners who have a combination of the right human qualities as well as the necessary knowledge and skills. If we are to deliver our vision this means workers who are open, honest, warm, empathetic and respectful, who treat people using services with equity, are non-judgemental and challenge unfair discrimination.

The workforce is therefore critical to delivery. We want to support all staff to move to a model which supports and promotes the independence of service users and carers. We are supporting initiatives in improving leadership and modernising the workforce and we are striving to find ways to improve the current workforce planning arrangements We are interested in views on how this could be achieved, and better integrated with the regional planning of Sector Skills Councils and across to the health sector.

WORKING WITH THE VOLUNTARY AND COMMUNITY SECTOR

Support for a strong and vibrant VCS is an essential component of our vision and developing the well-being agenda. We want to encourage and support community capacity-building at a local level. This will create opportunities for all citizens to contribute to society, to support people who may need assistance through volunteering, and to encourage the greater social inclusion of those who have traditionally been in receipt of help by giving them opportunities to contribute themselves.

We are playing an active role in helping the VCS to engage in participation locally with public sector commissioning authorities.

We also consider the wider issue of volunteering, including the development of time banks and other opportunities for mutual cooperation.

CONCLUSION

Independence, Well-being and Choice is intended to provoke discussion in order to hear your views on:

- how we can offer more control, more choice and high-quality support for those who use care services;
- how we can harness the capacity of the whole community, so that everyone has access to the full range of universal services and an opportunity to play a full part in society; and
- how we can improve the skills and status of the workforce to deliver the vision.

The key proposals to deliver this vision include:

- wider use of direct payments and the piloting of individual budgets to stimulate the development of modern services delivered in the way people want;
- greater focus on preventative services to allow for early, targeted interventions, and the use of the local authority well-being agenda to ensure greater social inclusion and improved quality of life;
- a strong strategic and leadership role for local government, working in partnership with other agencies, particularly the NHS, to ensure a wide range of effective and well-targeted provision, which meets the needs of our diverse communities; and
- encouraging the development of new and exciting models of service delivery and harnessing technology to deliver the right outcomes for adult social care.

We would now like to hear your views on our proposals so that together we can move forward by implementing a shared vision and creating a social care environment which is right for the 21st century.

PART ONE
Our vision for adult social care

1. Our vision for adult social care

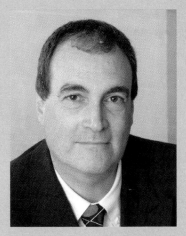

1.1 Our society is based on the belief that everyone has a contribution to make and has the right to control their own lives. This value drives our society and will also drive the way in which we provide social care.

1.2 This is a vision for all adults. It includes older people and younger adults who need care and support, people who are frail, people with a disability or mental health problems and people who care for or support other adults. It is also a vision for those who provide care services.

1.3 Services should be person-centred, seamless and proactive. They should support independence, not dependence and allow everyone to enjoy a good quality of life, including the ability to contribute fully to our communities. They should treat people with respect and dignity and support them in overcoming barriers to inclusion. They should be tailored to the religious, cultural and ethnic needs of individuals. They should focus on positive outcomes and well-being, and work proactively to include the most disadvantaged groups. We want to ensure that everyone, particularly people in the most excluded groups in our society, benefits from improvements in services.

1.4 Over the next 10 to 15 years, we want to work with people who use social care to help them transform their lives by:

- ensuring they have more control;
- giving them more choices and helping them decide how their needs can best be met;
- giving them the chance to do the things that other people take for granted; and
- giving the best quality of support and protection to those with the highest levels of need.

1.5 We will achieve this by:

- changing the ways social care services are designed. We will give people more control over them through self-assessment and through planning and management of their own services;
- developing new and innovative ways of supporting individuals;
- building and harnessing the capacity of the whole community to make sure that everyone has access to the full range of universal services; and
- improving the skills and status of the social care workforce.

1.6 In summary, the vision we have for social care services is one where:

- services help maintain the independence of the individual by giving them greater choice and control over the way in which their needs are met;
- the local authority and Director of Adult Social Services have key strategic and leadership roles and work with a range of partners, including primary care trusts and the independent and voluntary sectors, to provide services which are well planned and integrated, make the most effective use of available resources, and meet the needs of a diverse community;
- local authorities give high priority to the inclusion of all sections of the community and other agencies, including the NHS, recognise their own contribution to this agenda;
- services are of high quality and delivered by a well-trained workforce or by informal and family carers who are themselves supported;
- we make better use of technology to support people and provide a wide range of supported housing options;
- we provide services with an emphasis on preventing problems and ensure that social care and the NHS work on a shared agenda to help maintain the independence of individuals;

- people with the highest needs receive the support and protection needed to ensure their own well-being and the safety of society; and
- the risks of independence for individuals are shared with them and balanced openly against benefits.

1.7 We do not deliver this vision at the moment. Sadly, the organisation and provision of our services do not help everyone to meet these goals consistently.

1.8 We want to use this vision to demonstrate where we need to change and to guide the way we provide care. Our challenge is to make this vision a reality.

Dr Stephen Ladyman MP
Parliamentary Under Secretary
of State for Community

PART TWO
Setting the context

2. Why do we need a new vision?

SUMMARY

The Government's programme of reform of public services provides us with an opportunity to create a framework for social care that meets the requirements of the 21st century. Changes in population and communities mean that we are living longer, but are less likely to be part of a supportive, close-knit family. Communities are more diverse and existing services do not always recognise that. Society has higher expectations and people want greater control over their own lives and the risks they take. In future we will not have the workforce available to meet demands in traditional ways. Given the scale and nature of the changes, it is not acceptable to continue to deliver social care in the way we do today.

2.1 The Prime Minister has set out a challenging agenda for the reform of the public sector, and *Independence, Well-being and Choice* provides us with the opportunity to debate the nature of social care and develop an approach to social care that better fits the requirements of the 21st century.

"We are proposing to put an entirely different dynamic in place to drive our public services: one where the service will be driven not by the managers but by the user."

The Prime Minister, the Rt Hon Tony Blair MP, July 2004

2.2 The Prime Minister's vision demands that all public service providers, including providers of social care, seek to deliver personalised services that offer true choice, excellence and equality. Our

public services define what we want our society to be, and reflect its values and commitment to social justice and equity. We need good-quality social care and social services. A decent society should not only help those who need support to go about their lives; it must also support those who cannot look after themselves. In the modern world social care should provide this support, wherever possible, in a way that maintains the independence of the individual and leaves them in control.

2.3 Good services will not only improve the lives of the individuals involved, but will also have a positive impact on the well-being of the entire community. If adults who receive social care become more independent, they will have opportunities to contribute more. *Independence, Well-being and Choice* allows us:

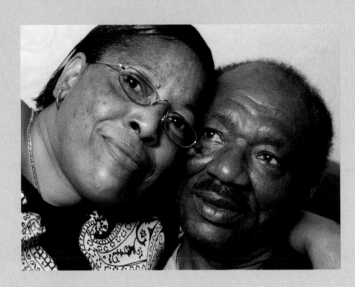

- an opportunity to set out our vision of the way that social care should develop over the next 10 to 15 years;
- to stimulate a wider debate about the values we expect within a modern, consumer-led public sector; and
- an opportunity to explore some of the mechanisms that might be used to bring about the changes that people who use services and carers tell us they want.

2.4 At the same time, our communities and population are changing. Many of us are living longer and we are less likely to be part of a close-knit family, who might have been there to support us in the past. This places increasing demands on formal services. We rightly expect our services, both public and private, to be of the highest quality, with the widest range of choice, and delivered in a way that leaves us in control of our lives. We cannot carry on delivering social care in the way we do today. It simply would not be acceptable to our communities.

CHANGES IN OUR LIVES: THE BALANCE OF RISK BETWEEN INDEPENDENCE AND PROTECTION

2.5 Today, society has higher expectations for prosperity, quality of life and standards of service than in the past. It is not just that people expect a higher quality of life, but that significantly more people expect it now than did in the past. This is progress. It is not the job of public services to tell people that they want too much. People do not want to be held back by their need for support. They tell us that they want services which help them maintain and develop their independence. These new expectations involve risk. We should now re-evaluate the range and type of services on offer and consider the balance between supporting people to manage risk in their lives and the need for protection at appropriate times.

CHANGES IN SOCIETY: DEVELOPING INDEPENDENCE IN A SOCIETY IN WHICH WE ARE MORE MOBILE

2.6 The proportion of people who live alone is likely to increase in the next 20 years because of increased longevity and changes in family structure. Our lives and those of our families involve much more geographical mobility than 50 years ago, and family and friends often have to cover large distances just to keep in touch, not only in this country but abroad. In fact, 21% of people over 65 see their family or friends less than once a week or not at all.[5] Increased mobility has broken some of the invisible strings that have traditionally bound families and communities. Mutual support becomes more difficult in these circumstances.

2.7 Our society is becoming more diverse and in many areas new communities have formed. Often we fail to respond with new, and differentiated, services that are appropriate to people's needs.

2.8 Changes in local economics have played a part in changing our society. The shifting focus away from the high street and towards out-of-town shopping centres and supermarkets has had a disproportionate effect on those who find it difficult to get around. In rural areas, families living on a low income can feel that limited local service provision and transport problems lead to isolation and social exclusion of a different nature from that of their town-dwelling counterparts. The closure of local shops, pubs and banks contributes to a sense of social decline. Living in a car-orientated society without a car can be a problem.[6]

CHANGES IN THE POPULATION: DEVELOPING INDEPENDENCE IN OUR SOCIETY

2.9 The change in the structure of our population is one of the most significant challenges we have to face in the 21st century.

2.10 There has been a long-term upward trend in the number of people aged 65 and over as life expectancy has increased considerably. In the last 100 years, the number of older people has increased by 400%. Since 1931, the number of older people has doubled.[7] Today, people over 100 years old are the fastest-growing group. This is a proud achievement which we are right to celebrate.

2.11 The latest population projections have predicted higher growth in the future than previously anticipated in the number of older people. The number of people over 65 is expected to rise over the next five decades from 9.3 million to 16.8 million. But the number of people over 85, the age group most likely to need nursing, residential or home care, is now expected to rise from 1.1 million in 2000 to 4 million in 2051.[8] However, future improvements in general health, or advances in the treatment of disabling illnesses

could lead to a reduction in the proportion of older people needing residential or nursing home care, making exact predictions of future demand difficult.

2.12 The population in rural areas is disproportionately affected by ageing. The evidence suggests that urban dwellers tend to migrate to rural areas on retirement. At the same time, younger people leave rural areas for career or educational reasons. This has resulted in a net shift of 780,000 people into rural areas between 1991 and 2001.[9]

2.13 It is estimated that as many as 800,000 people over the age of 20 have a learning disability. Assuming no changes to prevalence, and allowing for the predicted effects of the changing ethnic minority population, this figure is expected to rise by 14% to over 900,000 by 2021.[10] The number of people with severe learning disabilities may also increase by around 1% per annum for the next 15 years, with growing numbers of children and young people with complex disabilities surviving into adulthood.

2.14 The number of older people with mental health problems is growing rapidly. The number over 65 is predicted to rise by 10% in the next 10 years, and the greatest increase will be among those over 80. Depression is more common among older people, affecting between 10% and 16% of those over 65.[11] One-quarter of those over 85 develop dementia and one-third of these need constant care or supervision. There are currently over 700,000 people with dementia in the UK, and by 2040 it is estimated that this figure will be over 1.2 million.[12]

2.15 As many as one in six adults experience mental ill-health at some time in their life. The World Health Organization (WHO) predicts that depression will be the leading cause of disability by 2020. In addition, 13% of boys and 10% of girls between 11 and 15 have some form of mental disorder, and evidence suggests that the rates of mental health disorder among young people are increasing.[13]

2.16 The future size and composition of the population are the result of great strides made in improving the health of individuals, in public health and in material standards of life. However, after the post-war and 1960s 'baby booms' the birth rate fell, so the proportion of working to retired people will change substantially after the first quarter of this century, creating challenges for the future workforce.

2.17 The scale of change coming makes it vital for us to examine how social care can best meet these challenges. The need for social care will increase over the coming years. We therefore have to consider how we organise and deliver services and adopt new models to cope with both growing demand and workforce availability.

2.18 It is not realistic to plan to continue to deliver care in the way we have in the past. These challenges – the increased public expectation that people should be able to live with their own risk; increased geographical mobility, leading to the diminution of the support of the extended family; and the increased demand for organised social care – can only be met by reassessing the way in which social care is delivered.

3. Setting clear outcomes

SUMMARY

Care and support are provided as a community and are part of the core values of our society. Where support by family and friends is not enough, it is supplemented by more formal models offered by the statutory, independent and voluntary and community sectors. We propose clear outcomes for social care, derived from what people tell us they want. The outcomes will be used to test and challenge how far social care is moving towards delivering the vision.

WHAT IS SOCIAL CARE?

3.1 Most of us will at some point in our lives need support, whether for ourselves or on behalf of someone in our family, a friend or a neighbour. Often this care and support will be provided by family, friends and neighbours themselves and we should never forget the important contribution made by informal caring. Not only does it benefit those people who receive support: it benefits wider society and is a sign of the values we hold dear as a community.

The term **social care** is used to describe the wide range of services designed to support people in their daily lives and help them play a full part in society. It includes a range of practical services such as home care, day centres and residential and nursing homes. It can include practical assistance to help individuals overcome barriers to inclusion, such as supported entry into work for an individual with a mental health problem, a personal assistant to enable a disabled person to lead a full and active life or supporting a person with a learning disability to play a full part in their local community. It can include support in managing complex relationships and emotional distress. Social care includes those services directly commissioned by the local authorities and those services which an individual or family organise and commission themselves.

There are 150 local authorities across England with **social services** responsibilities, which have a statutory duty to assess the social care needs of individuals and to make arrangements for the provision of services to meet the needs of those people who are eligible for support. In planning and commissioning services, they have built partnerships with the NHS and with the independent, voluntary and community sectors. Evidence indicates that these partnerships need to be developed further.[14]

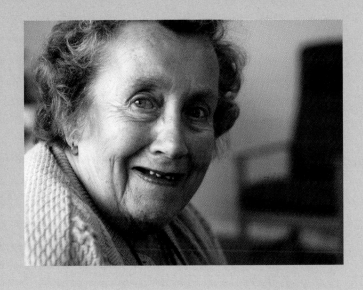

3.2 But sometimes informal care is not enough and cannot provide the level of support and service that is needed. This is when we turn to more formal models of social care and look to the statutory, independent, voluntary and community sectors to play their part. *Independence, Well-being and Choice* is concerned primarily with formal social care, while recognising that informal care is to be encouraged and promoted as part of the core values of our society.

SETTING CLEAR OUTCOMES FOR SOCIAL CARE

3.3 To turn the vision for adult social care into a reality we need to set clear outcomes for social care against which the experience of individuals can be measured and tested.

3.4 Since April 2004, we have held a nationwide dialogue on the future of adult social care. Independence, empowerment and choice have been the key themes to emerge.

3.5 To experience a good quality of life everyone needs to have independence, the ability to achieve their potential and the opportunity to participate fully in the life of their community. Of equal importance is the maintenance of positive relationships, respect and dignity.

3.6 The aims of adult social care must be appropriate for all adults, irrespective of age or need, including young people moving from children's to adults' services. We propose the outcomes outlined in the box overleaf as the basis of our framework for adult social care. They are central to the values upon which services should be built, and against which they should be tested. We will only achieve the vision if they are genuinely embedded in everything we do.

Improved health: enjoying good physical and mental health (including protection from abuse and exploitation). Access to appropriate treatment and support in managing long-term conditions independently. Opportunities for physical activity.

Improved quality of life: access to leisure, social activities and life-long learning and to universal, public and commercial services. Security at home, access to transport and confidence in safety outside the home.

Making a positive contribution: active participation in the community through employment or voluntary opportunities. Maintaining involvement in local activities and being involved in policy development and decision making.

Exercise of choice and control: through maximum independence and access to information. Being able to choose and control services. Managing risk in personal life.

Freedom from discrimination or harassment: equality of access to services. Not being subject to abuse.

Economic well-being: access to income and resources sufficient for a good diet, accommodation and participation in family and community life. Ability to meet costs arising from specific individual needs.

Personal dignity: keeping clean and comfortable. Enjoying a clean and orderly environment. Availability of appropriate personal care.

"People don't have high expectations, just to be treated with a bit of dignity and respect with some of the opportunities the rest of us take for granted."

"I've lost control of some things. I want control over my personal care."

"I wish there was somewhere to go during the day. I don't know about anywhere for people with multiple sclerosis to go in this area. It would give me something to talk about with my family, like going to work used to."

"Getting more help as a disabled parent with small children would be really helpful."

"The professionals really need to listen to the people who use services."

3.7 Few people will disagree with these outcomes, but delivering them will be challenging. Recent reports from the Commission for Social Care Inspection[15] suggest that there is some way to go before these themes are a reality in people's care.

Consultation questions

Your views are invited on the proposals set out in this chapter. In particular:

1. Does the vision for adult social care as set out summarise what social care for adults should be trying to achieve in the 21st century?
2. Are these the right outcomes for social care?

4. Putting people in control: improving assessment, direct payments and individual budgets

SUMMARY

We want to move to a system where adults are able to take greater control of their lives. We want to encourage a debate about risk management and the right balance between protecting individuals and enabling them to manage their own risks. We want to provide better information and signposting to allow people to retain responsibility and give people greater choice and control over how their needs should be met. We set out our proposals to increase the take-up of direct payments and to introduce individual budgets. We explain how these will enable individuals to make real choices.

4.1 For too long social work has been perceived as a gatekeeper or rationer of services, and has been accused, sometimes unfairly, of fostering dependence rather than independence. We want to create a different environment which reinforces the core social work values of supporting individuals to take control of their own lives and to make the choices which matter to them.

4.2 In order to do this, we want to move from a system where people have to take what is offered to one where people have greater control over identifying the type of support or help they want, and more choice about and influence over the services on offer. We plan to do this by giving everyone better information and signposting of services, putting people at the centre of the assessment process and creating individual budgets that give them greater freedom to select the type of care or support they want.

MANAGING RISKS

4.3 It is important to acknowledge that the proposals set out are not necessarily achievable in the same way for everyone across all areas of their lives and at all times. Risk is different for different people at different times of their lives and people have varying capacities to make their own judgements. Social care retains a responsibility for the protection of individuals, and we do not want to weaken the framework of protection that currently exists.

4.4 We know that many people who use social care place a high premium on autonomy. There is a balance to be struck between enabling people to have control over their lives and ensuring they are free from harm, exploitation and mistreatment, particularly if they cease to have the capacity to make informed choices. We believe that social workers and other professionals have difficult

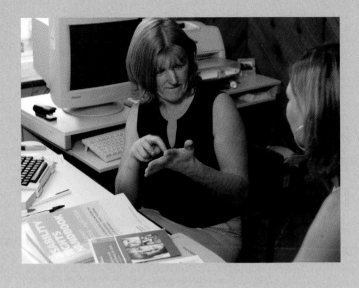

In the *No Secrets* guidance,[16] the Government has outlined a national framework placing a clear responsibility upon local authority social services to act as lead agencies in the development of local multi-agency codes of practice for the protection of vulnerable adults. The Government is also taking forward a programme of work to improve protection of this group in response to the recommendations of the Bichard Inquiry,[17] including the development of a registration scheme covering those working with vulnerable adults.

The primary responsibility for delivering quality services, including ensuring that people are safe from abuse and potential abuse, rests with local councils and with service providers. Inspectorates such as the Commission for Social Care Inspection (CSCI) also play an important role in ensuring that those charged with protecting people from harm do so.

judgements to make in seeking the right balance of protection for individuals from harm, and supporting them to understand and manage their own risks.

4.5 The greater appetite for people to retain more responsibility for their own life may at times conflict with the view of wider society and the media about the need to adopt a more protective stance. We would welcome a more open debate about risk management and what it means, which would enable social care staff to operate within a more supportive framework while meeting the legitimate aspirations of the people who use their services.

4.6 This will require a mechanism to 'protect' care assessors and care workers from blame when accidents occur. If risks are identified and a person using services understands and accepts them, then social workers must not be made scapegoats.

THE NEED FOR BETTER INFORMATION
4.7 Many of us recognise that we, or members of our family, have additional needs if we have a life-long disability or as we grow older and develop health problems. Despite these additional needs, we want solutions that remain within our own control, perhaps by identifying a service or piece of equipment ourselves. Often we are prevented from taking responsibility for what we need because of the difficulty of getting information on what support, help or equipment is available.

4.8 Information is clearly the key to decision making. Carers have also told us that they would like independent advice to enable them to make choices about their own lives and the options available to them. We would like councils to explore how they can provide better information which is easy to understand and is available in minority languages and a variety of formats, including easy read and braille or audio tapes. Other ways of providing information and advice that are sensitive to language and cultural needs should be developed. Better information can enable people to retain greater control over their lives and, where appropriate, take more responsibility for accessing the help and assistance they need. The Department of Health (DH) will also assess existing information and advice provision by 2006 and consider further steps.[18]

In August 2004, the Department for Work and Pensions (DWP) published *Link-Age: Developing networks of services for older people*. This promoted a vision that older people would have easy access in their local area to information about the full range of services available and builds on the lessons learnt from Care Direct. This model would be effective for all people who need support from social services. The key components are:

- easy access to advice and information;
- the promotion of neighbourliness and community support;
- better systems for sharing information between organisations; and
- ensuring that issues which matter to people using services are given proportionate weight in the community planning process.

Single point of access via the telephone
Somerset includes large rural areas, making it difficult for many older people to access information about services. The council provides a single telephone access point for all older people and their carers.

A customer rang to say she needed an occupational therapist to visit because she was having trouble getting in and out of the bath. At the same time, she was also helped to claim Attendance Allowance (AA), Pension Credit and Council Tax Benefit. She also obtained a blue badge helping her park near the shops. Her daughter was able to receive a Carer's Allowance. The package helped her to remain living independently in the community.

PUTTING PEOPLE AT THE CENTRE OF ASSESSMENT

4.9 Where an individual is unable to access the support they require or their needs are more complex, social services will be involved in their assessment. The traditional way in which services have been provided has been through an assessment of an individual by a social care worker. This model works well where the relationship allows for a full discussion within which genuine choice can be promoted. However, difficulties such as shortage of staff or resources, problems with communication or a power imbalance in the relationship can lead to outcomes that may not genuinely address the individual's needs, or enable the person using care to exercise genuine choice.

4.10 In some cases, people have been assessed, only to be told that the support they need is not available locally, or that it is outside the range of services that the local authority has chosen to fund.

4.11 There must be a better approach that puts people using services and carers at the centre of needs assessment, allows people to take more responsibility, and frees social workers to use their skills to achieve better outcomes for those who need greatest support. We must also challenge the approach that the services offered are those that are available and not those that the individual would choose.

4.12 Some people may be able to benefit from self-assessment by identifying, for example, minor adaptations and equipment, freeing up scarce occupational therapy resources for those who have more complex needs. Kent County Council is pioneering a new, interactive self-assessment website to offer this.

> **Self-assessment using the internet**
> The new site, www.kent.gov.uk/selfassessment, is available to all residents over 18, and enables people to interact with social services staff, and select the level of service which best fits their needs.
>
> It means, for example, that for the first time, people with moderate needs are given a fast, round-the-clock decision about whether they qualify for support. Carers or relatives are also able to fill out the user-friendly form on behalf of someone else, effectively enabling someone in Melbourne to complete an assessment on behalf of an older parent in Maidstone. Anyone assessed as eligible for help will be offered the choice of using direct payments to arrange services themselves and control the whole process.

4.13 Others may not have access to self-assessment tools or not want to use them: many people will want support. It is also the case that a significant number of people currently supported by social services have complex needs or severe mental health needs which may limit their ability to assess their own requirements and manage their own risks. For everyone undergoing an assessment, whether the person using services or their carer, the starting assumption should be that they have the capacity to express views and wishes. Support should be put in place, and time taken to enable people to choose how they want to be supported.

Their views and wishes should form the starting point of assessment undertaken by a skilled professional within a multidisciplinary approach, which itself retains the principle that the individual should be at the heart of the assessment and should be able to make their own choices where they have the capacity to do so.

4.14 In developing support arrangements, account should be taken of specific local needs and circumstances in the development of culturally sensitive services. It is likely over the coming years that the proportion of older, frail people from different ethnic groups will change. For example, the demographics of immigration from the Caribbean, Africa and South Asia since the war means that there will be increasing numbers of older people from black and ethnic minority groups over the coming years. Patterns of immigration from other parts of the world in recent years mean that cultural needs are likely to continue to change in the future.

4.15 In addition, people with complex needs cannot be considered in isolation from the families or the communities in which they live. Adults with dementia, complex mental health problems or disabilities have a considerable impact on families, friends and carers. Only by taking account of their needs, the needs of the whole family and responsibilities of family members, including those for dependent children and young people, will it be possible to identify what services or interventions are needed.

4.16 Of course, the individual's own assessment of their needs might conflict with those of their professional assessor. At present, this is too often hidden. The individual's personal assessment must be transparent in this whole process. That is what happens in the rest of our lives. We work out what we want and then, in trying to achieve it, we may have to negotiate because of limits to resources or other factors.

A young woman, Claire, had been living in a registered care home for some time. She didn't get on well with the other residents and she found it difficult to communicate with them. She didn't like living in a large group. She was asked to leave because she was 'too difficult to support in the home'.

She lived temporarily in a respite care service but this arrangement also broke down. She had to move a long way away from her family for her new service, which she found very upsetting. Fortunately her family, helped by a circle of support, were able to work out, with Claire, some ideas about where and how she wanted to live.

They found a housing provider, Advance, who operate a shared ownership scheme, allowing people to buy a share of a property. The housing provider remains involved and retains responsibility for repairs and maintenance. Using this scheme, a suitable property was found for Claire on the south coast where she could be closer to her family.

A separate support provider was also identified to support Claire on a person-centred basis. This support is arranged through direct payments.

She is now in control of her home and the support that she receives.

THE 'RIGHT TO REQUEST'

4.17 As part of our wider consultation about how people are supported in expressing their needs through the assessment process, we have decided to consult specifically on the merits of a 'right to request' not to live in a residential or nursing care setting, taking full account of the particular issues faced by the individual, and considering the financial, organisational and legal implications of both the status quo and alternative options. This 'right to request' would require service providers to make explicit the reasons behind their decision to recommend residential care, including cost considerations. This information would support the

individual to make informed choices about options available to them. In consulting on this, we are following the recommendations in the Prime Minister's Strategy Unit report *Improving the Life Chances of Disabled People.*[19] We welcome your views on this recommendation.

IMPROVING ASSESSMENT

4.18 We already have models for multidisciplinary assessments for the provision and review of services in the single assessment process (SAP)[20] and care programme approach (CPA)[21] for people with severe and enduring mental illness. We also have *Valuing People's*[22] expectation that people with learning disabilities are supported to develop their own person-centred plan, the achievement of those aspirations being an objective of professional assessments. The introduction of the long-term conditions model[23] and the role of community matrons[24] also provides us with an opportunity to look again at how an individual can be supported to identify needs and obtain the appropriate range of services.

4.19 While skilled social work is not essential for all assessments, we expect it to continue to be key in:

- the assessment of needs for people with complex problems and where there is a significant impact on families and carers including children and young people in the family. The need for skilled social work is **not** to replace the views of the person who needs care; the skill is to find out what people themselves want;
- the development of constructive relationships and specific therapeutic interventions to assist people needing long-term support for themselves and in their roles within families as parents and carers;
- coordinating services and negotiating systems to meet complex needs and maintain positive outcomes; and
- assessing risk to individuals and to the community.

STREAMLINING ASSESSMENT ACROSS AGENCIES

4.20 We are interested in ways of providing a better service for people who are eligible for support through the local authority and other agencies. These people may also be entitled to AA or Disability Living Allowance (DLA). These are DWP benefits which are paid as a contribution towards the extra costs faced by people with severe disabilities because of those disabilities. They are claimed mainly on the basis of self-assessed personal care needs and, in the case of DLA, walking difficulties. Individuals also have to provide information, for example about their care and housing needs when seeking support from the local authority. We would like to explore the extent to which the need for people to provide broadly the same information to more than one agency could be minimised. This might be achieved through DWP and local authorities sharing information provided in connection with AA/DLA claims and from overview assessments between health and social care. We will seek to experiment with more streamlined assessments including self-assessment, as discussed earlier, covering a wider range of other budgets.

GIVING PEOPLE THE MEANS TO CHOOSE: DIRECT PAYMENTS AND INDIVIDUAL BUDGETS

4.21 People at the centre of assessment have the opportunity to choose what services and support they think would best meet their needs. The services and support chosen might be different from the services that the formal care system has on offer, and we want to create a mechanism that will allow individuals to keep control and choice over their situation and the support they actually receive.

4.22 In talking to people who use services and to carers, it is clear that direct payments[25] give people that choice and control, and we think that this is a mechanism that should be extended and encouraged where possible.

> Taking control of his own support arrangements allowed Mr Clarke to go on a fishing trip, accompanied by his assistant, while his wife took a break from her caring role and went on holiday. Mr Clarke paid £100 for three nights away and 24-hour assistance, paying extra from his own pocket to cover the costs. He said this was much more enjoyable, and cheaper, than institutional respite care: "It's brilliant."[26]

4.23 Take up of direct payments has so far been disappointing. There are 12,585 individuals in receipt of direct payments (provisional 2003 estimate).[27] By contrast there were 1.68 million adults using community care services in 2002/03. We would therefore like to encourage more people to consider whether direct payments are right for them, particularly in groups where take-up has been low, such as older people, people with mental health problems and young people moving to adult services.

4.24 We also want to consider ways of extending the benefits of direct payments to those currently excluded, by using an agent for those without the capacity to consent, or unable to manage even with assistance. This means, for example, that a child who currently has direct payments managed by a parent could continue to receive direct payments after the age of 18, even if they have a disability so severe they cannot give consent for themselves. More details of these proposals can be found at Appendix C and we welcome views on them.

INDIVIDUAL BUDGETS

4.25 We think that all groups have the potential to benefit from the opportunity to have greater control over the services they need and how these should be provided, in a way that offers the real benefit of choice and control of direct payments, without the potential burdens.

4.26 We are already testing a new approach through the In Control[28] pilots for people with learning disabilities. In Control is a national programme in England to promote a self-directed support approach to social care. It is funded by local authorities and Mencap and supported by the Valuing People Support Team. It is running in six local authority test sites in Essex, Gateshead, Redcar, South Gloucestershire, West Sussex and Wigan. Early results from these sites have given us some very encouraging case studies of how a more person-centred and transparent allocation of social care funds can transform the quality of life of people with learning disabilities.

4.27 We know that our ability to increase the number of people who can take advantage of direct payments is limited by the barriers that some people experience in taking them up. Currently a person using services has legal responsibilities for someone they employ through direct payments. They may also take on the risk of recruitment. In some cases they would have to organise payroll, National Insurance contributions and a number of other statutory employer responsibilities. This is a considerable responsibility that many individuals, especially older people, may find burdensome.[29]

4.28 Therefore, building on the model of the In Control pilots for people with learning disabilities, and on the recommendations of the Prime Minister's Strategy Unit report *Improving the Life Chances of Disabled People,*[30] we propose to test the introduction of 'individual budgets' for adults with a disability or with an assessed need for social care support.

4.29 The purpose of an individual budget would be to promote independent living. This is not just about being able to stay in your own home but is also about providing people with choice, empowerment and freedom. This new approach is about allocating available resources according to individual needs, in the form of individual budgets made transparent to the person requiring services. The budget would be held by the local authority

on behalf of the person using services or their carer. People could have individual support to identify the services they wish to use, which might be outside the range of services traditionally offered by social care.

4.30 Individuals should be able to choose whether they receive support in the form of a cash direct payment or provision of services. Either way, the budget should be used to secure the appropriate type of support for the individual. For those who choose not to take a direct payment as cash, the budgets would give many of the benefits of choice to the person using services without them having the worry of actually managing the money for themselves.

4.31 This new approach would require radical changes to the way in which budgets are organised and services are delivered. The options for a new system to deliver this approach should be piloted and people using services will need to be at the heart of these pilots.

4.32 Therefore, DH will, supported by other government departments, develop an evidence base for individual budgets through the creation of a number of pilots. The pilots will work with different groups of adults, looking at a range of different approaches working within existing resources and with local organisations that have already made progress in this area. Subject to the success of the pilots and the availability of new resources to initiate change, individual budgets could be introduced for people with a disability by 2012.

4.33 Individual budgets could be used solely for social care (to replace or co-exist with current direct payments). However, high levels of bureaucracy, repetitive assessments and piecemeal approaches to meeting individual needs indicate that extending the scope of individual budgets to closely allied services would benefit the individual.

4.34 We will also consider whether a range of other budgets, for example community care resources and social services expenditure on minor equipment and adaptations, Independent Living Funds, Access to Work and Family Funds should also be included and test this, where appropriate, through pilots working in conjunction with colleagues from other government departments including DWP.

4.35 Giving people an individual budget should drive up the quality of services. The ability of people to 'buy' elements of their care or support package will stimulate the social care market to provide the services people actually want, and help shift resources away from services which do not meet needs and expectations. We intend that the introduction of individual budgets will help promote the more effective use of the resources available to meet care needs.

4.36 By giving people an individual budget to buy services of their own choosing, we are giving them a greater opportunity to identify where services fail to meet their needs or the outcomes their vision demands. They will be able to transfer that share of the budget into something more appropriate. In so doing, we can create opportunities to quality control existing services and develop new and more flexible service models which meet needs, for example, in a more culturally sensitive way, or in a location more suitable for a rural population. People who are currently the passive recipients of services become consumers with the ability to shape and control the services they are willing to buy and shift the culture of care planning.

4.37 People using direct payments can, at present, buy services from any provider but not from a direct care department of a local council. They can choose to receive a mixture of direct care and direct payments, but some councils tell us they would like people to be able to take all their care through direct payments and 'buy' services from the council. Introducing individual budgets would allow this sort of flexibility and provide an incentive for councils to match standards in the private sector and vice versa.

4.38 We believe that the needs assessment and the estimate of an individual budget should be done before a financial assessment is undertaken. Only after the needs have been assessed should there be a discussion about the level of private contribution to be made to the cost of provision.

4.39 Clearly, the development of individual budgets will present a number of potential models, which will require further development and piloting so that we can be confident that further expansion will deliver the choice, empowerment and better use of resources we seek. We would particularly welcome views on the piloting and development of individual budgets.

4.40 In order to put people at the centre of assessment and give them individual budgets, many will need help and support to clarify their views on the support they want and to access the services they need. This includes those people who will have to pay for some or all of their support from their own funds. A number of models have been suggested and we would like to explore the range of options further, to identify the most promising and cost-effective means of providing support.

A **person-centred planning facilitator** to support the person to develop their own aspirations as the basis for future service plans.

A **care manager** working alongside the person who may need services to undertake the needs assessment and act as lead professional to case manage the care package. This model might be particularly valuable to support those with very complex needs and provide continuity of skilled social work input. The role might also be undertaken by another professional as part of the multidisciplinary team, for example a community matron.

A **care navigator** with knowledge of mainstream and specialist services, working with the person using services to develop a sustained pathway of care.

A **care broker** who might help the individual formulate the care plan, negotiate funding and help organise and monitor services.

4.41 Whoever performs the role of supporting individuals through the system will need to be knowledgeable about what is available, what different agencies or services beyond social services can offer, and how people's aspirations for themselves can be turned into reality. Even more important than that knowledge is the skill in supporting the independence of the individual receiving care. These tasks must empower people to live the lives they want by, for example, supporting them back into employment, helping to overcome the multiple problems associated with homelessness, or finding the right services to enable an older person to stay at home.

Consultation questions

Views are invited on the proposals set out in this chapter. In particular:

3. What are your views about how we can strike an appropriate balance in managing risks between individuals, the community and the social care worker?

4. Should we take forward proposals to minimise the need for people to provide broadly the same information, for instance by sharing information between agencies such as the local authority and DWP?

5. We welcome views on modernising assessment and putting individuals at its centre. We are particularly interested in the practicalities of self-assessment. Do you think that there should be professional social work involvement in some or all assessments?

6. Do you have views on whether the SAP, the CPA and person-centred planning (PCP) should be further developed to provide a tool for use with all people with complex needs?

7. How can we encourage greater take-up of direct payments in under-represented groups such as older people and people with mental health problems?

8. Extending the scope of direct payments (see Appendix C for more details).
    i.   Do you think we should review the exclusions under the direct payments regulations?
    ii. Do you think that extending direct payments should initially be a power or a duty for local councils?
    iii. What do you think about the proposal to extend direct payments via an agent to groups currently excluded, namely those unable to give consent or manage a payment, even with assistance?

9. Changing the name of direct payments (see Appendix D for more details).
    i.   Which name for direct payments is the most appropriate? Are there any others?
    ii. When do you think the change should be introduced?

10. We are committed to the introduction of individual budgets to give people greater control over their lives. We would welcome views on the proposals to pilot individual budgets.

11. We are proposing to introduce a care navigator/broker model and would welcome views on these proposals. What are your views on the skills needed to perform the function and whether such a model might free social worker expertise to deal with the most complex cases?

5. The role of the wider community

SUMMARY

We emphasise the importance of carers and their role in this vision. We also discuss how we can extend the range of choice and make links with the local authority well-being agenda.

THE ROLE OF CARERS

5.1 Many people with significant needs receive care from relatives or friends. These relationships are vital to our communities. The Government has already introduced a number of measures that recognise the vital role that carers play. The Carers (Equal Opportunities) Act 2004 was established to ensure that carers are able to take up opportunities that those without caring responsibilities take for granted.

5.2 The key to supporting carers in undertaking their vital role is to provide the right level of support for them, which enables them to make choices about their personal life. In providing support and services for carers, local authorities should adopt the approach set out in our vision. Carers should be supported to decide how their needs should be met through full involvement in their assessment.

5.3 Carers also tell us that they would like access to training and support in their caring role. Not only would this improve the quality of the experience for the person receiving care, it might

also offer the carer who has left employment a longer-term route into education and training, and into more formal paid employment once their immediate caring responsibilities cease. We believe that this should form part of any local workforce development initiative and would expect it to be considered by every local workforce development strategy.

EXTENDING THE RANGE OF SUPPORT

5.4 If we take the vision and the outcomes at all seriously as real goals rather than just words, we have to challenge our assumptions about how support is delivered, and how social services departments can harness and foster the other resources that already exist in the local community. This is particularly true in areas with diverse populations. We want to link social care more strongly to the wider well-being agenda of local authorities, build on the well-being focus promoted by *Choosing Health*,[31] and offer services and support which prevent individuals becoming dependent and needing more specialised social care interventions.

5.5 People who use services, and their carers, tell us that the service or support that would make a real difference to their lives is often one that is not available through local social services departments. We want to change that. We want to encourage the care manager or care navigator to work with the individual to identify ways in which those needs can be met, and to be more flexible in looking at the overall balance of needs and services. For example, a carer might be willing to take on additional caring responsibilities in return for more help with some routine domestic chores, and an older person might prefer to meet a friend rather than attend a lunch club if accessible public transport were available.

5.6 Not all of the costs of offering wider and more flexible packages fall within social services department budgets. We want to encourage a more flexible approach to putting together packages using the wider resources of the community. A package could include a mixture of more traditional social care items, use of universal services already provided by the local authority, and a contribution from the local voluntary and community sector.

5.7 By definition, universal services should be designed to enable all members of the community to have access. They include, among others, education and health, libraries, leisure facilities and transport. They can provide a valuable contribution to the wider well-being agenda. Too often, for many people currently using social care, the existing models of universal services are such as to prevent them gaining access to the very services the rest of us take for granted. For example, people with a mental health problem may be prevented from accessing education; leisure services may not be available for those with a disability; and an older person's ability to get around may be hampered by inaccessible forms of transport. We want to encourage those who provide universal services to make them accessible to everyone in the community.

5.8 Transport and leisure services are obvious examples of services that contribute to the well-being and prevention agenda by fostering independence and social inclusion, but others, such as planning and design, can also play their part in improving access and inclusion for people with disabilities and for older people. Disabled access to streetscapes and public areas, transport and community safety designed around the needs of this group, and the design of housing to accommodate people with particular needs, are all areas where mainstream services can make a contribution to overall well-being and reduce the need for more specialist social services.

> "Design for the young and you exclude the old; design for the old and you include the young."
>
> **Professor Bernard Isaacs (1924–1995)**

ENCOURAGING PREVENTATIVE SERVICES

5.9 In future, greater focus should be placed on preventative services through the wider well-being agenda and through better targeted, early interventions that prevent or defer the need for more costly intensive support. Current eligibility criteria allow for early intervention and support. More use of universal services could help people remain better integrated in their communities, prevent social isolation and maintain independence. This will allow social care to play its specialist and essential role in supporting those with specific needs that cannot be met in this way.

6. Funding and fair access to care

SUMMARY

This chapter sets out the scale of social care spending; recognises that implementing the vision will need to be managed within the existing funding envelope; and identifies scope for making better use of funding. It raises questions about how the proposals set out in the vision tie in with Fair Access to Care Services (FACS) and seeks views.

FUNDING

6.1 Social care is big business. Approximately £14.4 billion of public funds will be invested in social care in England in 2004/05, of which £10.6 billion is for services for adults. Investment in personal social services will be £1.8 billion higher by 2007/08 representing an annual average increase of 2.7% in real terms above that of 2004/05.

6.2 Coupled with this significant public investment in social care is the important contribution of those who pay for services themselves. An estimated 30% of adults pay for their own residential care. Other social care services are means-tested in most areas and subject to contributions from those with income and assets that exceed certain thresholds.

6.3 The changes proposed in *Independence, Well-being and Choice* will need to be met from existing funds. That is why we have suggested that this is a vision for the next 10 to 15 years. We know that change of this order cannot be introduced overnight and that local organisations will need

time to manage the transition required for the introduction of individual budgets and greater choice for those who need support.

6.4 We recognise that some resources are tied up in unnecessary assessments, or in services that may no longer best meet the needs and requirements of people using services today. We are keen to look at alternative models, which will deliver the desired outcomes, which might allow resources to be diverted to areas that are currently less well supported.

6.5 It is clear that, if we make better use of the funding we have available across the system, we can free up resources to improve quality and capacity. We want to use all the resources available in the system to deliver the services that meet people's needs. In some cases, the flexibilities of the 1999 Health Act[32] and the 2000 Local Government Act[33] have been used to deliver better quality, targeted services to those who need them in a more cost-effective way. We want to explore

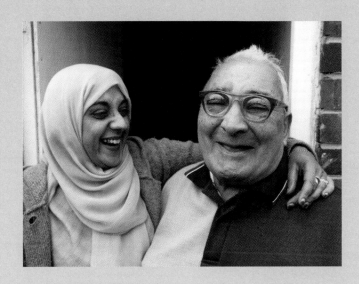

the extension of such models to deliver benefits to greater numbers of people.

6.6 The review undertaken by Sir Peter Gershon[34] suggests that efficiency savings can be made by rationalising back-office functions, procurement and transactional services, the development of effective, evidence-based policy and focused inspection and regulation. The review has led to a target for efficiency savings of 2.5% across local government services.

The Department of Health (DH) has set up the care services efficiency programme seeking to make savings of £228 million in 2005/06 rising to £684 million in 2007/08. The programme team has already begun developing an efficiency excellence framework with local councils, where improvement in service quality is central to the framework, and will be reporting its recommendations in the first half of 2005.

6.7 Savings made through this programme and the Gershon Review are to be reinvested in services for communities. Effective procurement should not be in conflict with giving greater choice to individuals through individual budgets. Improved strategic commissioning should deliver both efficiency gains and the right balance, range and quality of services to meet local needs. The Government will explore

how to support councils to improve their strategic commissioning.

6.8 The care services efficiency programme is looking at a number of processes, including the scope for the reduction of unnecessary bureaucracy. We will be feeding the results of the review into the development of pilots. Colleagues directly responsible for services will be closely involved in the development of these pilots.

FAIR ACCESS TO CARE

6.9 Giving people greater control over how their needs are met and the services they require raises genuine concerns about whether greater pressures will be placed on existing budgets. There is some evidence from direct payments and In Control pilots that indicates that needs can be met, in more cost-efficient ways, if the support is available in the way the individual wants.[35] The end result may then be less expensive than the traditionally assessed package of care.

6.10 There is also evidence[36] that if older people, those with learning disabilities or sensory impairment in particular, can access relatively inexpensive adaptations or pieces of equipment at an early stage, they can defer or avoid the need for more significant interventions by social services or the NHS. When people with mental health problems are supported effectively in the community, they may remain well. More costly health and social care interventions could be prevented by harnessing the resources of universal services and the voluntary and community sector more effectively to deliver a broader package of care.

6.11 Shifting the balance of services from high-level needs to earlier, preventative interventions will have implications not only for managing the budget but also for the existing eligibility criteria, their application and the way in which local councils determine who should be eligible for services. It will be important to continue to develop the evidence base for this approach to identify cost-effective solutions. Clear policies and protocols on the way in which different social service teams and units for all groups work together will be required, if we are to avoid an unnecessary fragmentation of services. This is particularly true where children and families teams are working alongside adult teams to ensure the specific needs of children and adults are both addressed and to recognise that assistance to a parent is often the most effective means of promoting the welfare of the child.

6.12 *Fair Access to Care Services*[37] provides guidance from DH to assist in deciding who should receive social care services from statutory agencies. FACS provides a framework that determines how councils should carry out assessments and reviews, and provide or commission services to meet needs, subject to available resources.

6.13 We believe that local authorities must retain the right to set local priorities and manage their budget and that those who approach the local authority should know that funding decisions are made on the basis of clearly understood criteria. We would therefore welcome views on the continued existence of FACS and how eligibility criteria can be set up to encompass both higher levels of need and early intervention.

6.14 We expect that overall the proposals in this Green Paper will be cost-neutral for local authorities. However, in developing any detailed proposals as a result of this consultation, DH will look closely at the cost implications for individual local authorities taking into account our commitment to the New Burdens Doctrine.[38]

Consultation question

Your views are invited on the proposals set out in this chapter. In particular:

12. What do you think will be the impact of shifting the balance of services from high-level need to earlier, preventative interventions on the eligibility criteria and what this might mean for FACS?

PART THREE
Creating the right environment

7. The strategic and leadership role of local government

SUMMARY

This chapter highlights the important leadership role played by local government, in particular by the Director of Adult Social Services (DASS). It suggests the development of a needs assessment and highlights the responsibility for managing the social care market.

LEADERSHIP

7.1 To deliver the change in focus and improved services, and to develop the necessary strategic approach, high-quality leadership will be essential at both officer and member level in local authorities. We are undertaking a separate consultation exercise which explores this in more detail.

7.2 The introduction of the post of DASS alongside the Director of Children's Services will ensure that all the social care needs of local communities are given equal emphasis and are managed in a coordinated way. The relationship between these two posts will be crucial to ensuring that the needs of both adults and children in families are met and that services work well together.

7.3 The development of the role of the DASS forms an essential part of our vision for the future of adult social care. We expect that each DASS will have seven key roles:

- providing accountability for spending on social care and delivering quality services;
- providing professional leadership for the social care workforce and championing the rights of adults with social care needs in the wider community;
- leading the implementation of standards to drive up the quality of care;
- managing a process of cultural change to implement proactive, seamless and person-centred services;
- promoting local access and ownership and driving forward partnership working to deliver a responsive, whole-system approach to social care;
- delivering an integrated approach to supporting communities by working closely with the Director of Children's Services to support individuals with care needs through the different stages of their lives; and
- promoting social inclusion and well-being to deliver a proactive approach to meeting the care needs of adults in culturally sensitive ways.

7.4 Our aim is to move to a position where there is clear accountability and an integrated strategy for adult social care both locally and nationally and a clear focus on the care needs of adults. We are simultaneously publishing best practice guidance on the role of the DASS for consultation. This guidance forms an integral part of our vision for the future of adult social care. The guidance can be found on the internet at www.dh.gov.uk/consultations.

NEEDS ASSESSMENT AND MARKET MANAGEMENT

7.5 Involving people in designing services to meet their individual needs brings new challenges. We have to ensure there is enough capacity to support the increasing demand for the range of options to be available. Supporting and developing wider market capacity and commissioning services at a more strategic level is essential. We suggest that the DASS and local authority should undertake regular strategic needs assessments to plan ahead for the next 10 to 15 years. These assessments should include consideration of the care and support needs of the whole population, including those who have the ability to pay for services themselves, and reflect the increased levels of joint working between health and social care and other service providers.

7.6 The needs assessment should be publicly available. It should give independent and voluntary sector providers more scope to plan for the future and develop a longer-term relationship with the commissioners of services. We recognise that most care is now provided by these sectors. The assessment would enable them to invest in services to meet the expanding needs of the 'self-funded' market, where services are not directly commissioned by local authorities. A healthy range of providers offering diversity and good-quality services will make individual choice a reality. Local authorities have an important role in promoting the development of the market. The Government will explore how best to support local authorities in

carrying out this role. We need to find innovative ways in which they can work with people, regardless of whether or not they need local authority help to access services, and with providers to achieve the outcomes people want.

7.7 The local needs assessment should be linked with the wider assessment of housing need in the area, which must encompass the housing needs of older people and those with disabilities and which underpins the local or sub-regional housing strategy. If people are to be supported to live at home in greater numbers, we need to make sure that local housing stock is suitable, in terms of condition and adaptability and that we make best use of adapted housing stock already in the system. The new Regional Housing Boards have been tasked to draw up regional housing plans which will take account of the need to promote and maintain the independence of people to help them stay in their own homes.[39]

Consultation questions

Your views are invited on the proposals set out in this chapter. In particular:

13. What is the best approach to strengthening leadership at council member level?
14. Do you support the introduction of a strategic needs assessment to inform the development of the social care market?
15. How can local authorities stimulate the market to offer a range and diversity of provision which meets the outcomes demanded by the vision?

We are consulting separately on the role of the DASS. Details of this consultation can be found on the internet at www.dh.gov.uk/consultations.

8. Shifting the focus of services: strategic commissioning

SUMMARY

This chapter recognises the need to develop a strategic commissioning framework with partners, to ensure the right balance between prevention, meeting low-level needs and providing intensive care and support for those with high-level complex needs. We also explore mechanisms for strengthening collaborative and partnership working.

8.1 In the last decade, social services and the NHS have increasingly concentrated resources on people with the highest levels of need. Consequently there has been less investment in promoting the health, independence and well-being of the general adult population. This has resulted in a less proactive approach to identifying and responding to needs as they emerge. Changing the focus to a preventative model of care by targeting people with low-level needs today, could prevent them from becoming part of the group of people with 'greatest needs' in the future.

8.2 There is a small but growing evidence base indicating significant potential benefits in low-level prevention aimed at improving well-being, and involving the range of local council services such as housing, transport, leisure and community safety, in addition to social care.[40] Social care services can also help to prevent inappropriate use of specialist healthcare. For example, too many older people are admitted to hospital, often as an emergency, when this could be avoided if the right community services were in place.[41]

8.3 Social care services can be effective, not only in preventing unnecessary admissions but also in reducing episodes of delayed discharge from hospital. We have already seen very significant reductions in the numbers of people delayed and much of this improvement has resulted from good joint working between health and social care partners. In addition, we know that well-timed interventions and greater social inclusion can prevent or reduce the severity of episodes of mental illness.

8.4 To achieve the vision and its outcomes, local partners will need to work together to promote and ensure a strategic balance of investment in local services for:

- the general population, aimed at promoting health and social inclusion;
- people with emerging needs, to provide support to enable them to maintain their independence; and

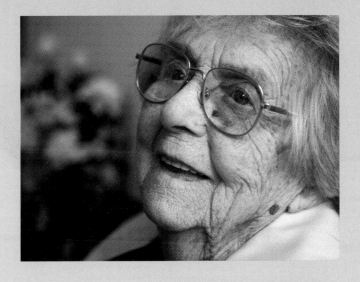

● those with high-level complex needs, to provide intensive care and support.

8.5 Local partners will need to recognise the diversity of their local communities and ensure that there is a range of services, which meet the needs of all members of the local community.

8.6 We are keen to encourage a shift to prevention and integrated delivery across health and social care. To support this we are investing £60 million over the years 2006/07 and 2007/08 to set up joint projects between councils and their NHS and local government partners to provide seamless integrated care for older people and to encourage investment in preventative services. Partnerships for Older People Projects[42] will test approaches to establishing sustainable arrangements for preventative services.

8.7 We therefore suggest that a local strategic commissioning framework should be developed with a range of partners and should cover the following:

● **Community development, social capital and inclusion, by:**
  – building community capacity through supporting the local voluntary and community sector (VCS) and developing local community volunteering strategies;
  – improving access to universal services; and

  – providing access to good-quality and affordable housing.

● **Prevention, enablement and early intervention services, including:**
  – adapted or specialist housing services;
  – health promotion;
  – improved prevention services, eg to prevent falls;
  – employment, training and access schemes;
  – early intervention services and better information and advice, eg Link-Age services to support benefits take-up and better knowledge of local services; and
  – telecare and preventative electronic technology.

● **Support and care services:**
  – built around self-assessment and the promotion of individual independence and choice, delivered through clear integrated pathways to which specialist services contribute;
  – frameworks for the protection of individuals;
  – crisis and assertive outreach services;
  – intensive, high-need and long-term care; and
  – diversity of provision.

● **Collaborative partnerships:**
  – joint commissioning with other authorities, the NHS, the VCS and people using services, to design and deliver seamless services.

IMPROVING INTEGRATED PARTNERSHIP WORKING

8.8 Across the country, there are some good examples of close working between agencies, but we need to do more to remove barriers to reaching an understanding of shared objectives and priorities. These will also need to reflect key policy initiatives such as the National Service Frameworks (NSFs) and the *Choosing Health* White Paper. Only agreement on the necessity for joined-up working will deliver a wholesale move to strategic, integrated services for the whole community

8.9 Many of the issues discussed in this paper are ones that the Government is considering more widely as part of the development of a 10-year strategy for local government.[43] In particular the Government intends to issue further discussion papers covering service delivery and the performance framework in the coming months.

8.10 The provisions of the Local Government Act 2000 facilitate closer working across local council services and beyond, and local communities are already seeing the benefits of local strategic partnerships (LSPs).[44] We now need to explore further ways to encourage local communities to provide social care in a way that recognises the complexity of delivery across a number of agencies.

8.11 Local area agreements[45] (LAAs) provide an opportunity for government, a local authority and its partners to improve public services by agreeing the design and delivery of outcome targets which reflect national and local priorities. They will enable partners to bring together the range of diverse funding streams at a local level, creating greater flexibility and efficiency. Local Public Service Agreements (LPSAs) can offer the incentive of a reward for achieving extra improvement beyond what would have been expected anyway. The rewards can be used by the partnership as they choose. In LAA areas, LPSAs sit alongside the LAA as part of a whole Agreement.

8.12 Improved partnership working has also been facilitated by provision for pooling of health and social care budgets in the Health Act 1999. Pooled budgets and integrated funding provide the flexibility for funds to flow to where they are most needed, in order to provide a truly personalised service. Successful programmes using these flexibilities have already demonstrated a shift away from high-intensity specialist care to lower-level, often preventative services.

As part of the Innovation Forum, 10 councils have set up strategic partnerships with their NHS partners to develop community services for older people which will reduce the number of emergency bed days for local people over 75 by 20% over three years.

One such partnership is the Edith Summerskill Unit run by Harlow Primary Care Trust and Hertfordshire County Council with the aim of helping and encouraging people to regain their independence or become as independent as possible. It is not a care home, but offers a setting for those who no longer need to be in hospital but are not ready to go home or who, if the unit was not available, might have had to be admitted to hospital. The care is provided by a multidisciplinary team of nursing and care staff, social workers, and therapists, who provide active support to help people regain strength, independence and confidence to return home.

8.13 Improved partnership working can also help to provide better access to services. Local transport authorities have been asked to work with their partners to produce accessibility strategies as part of their next local transport plans. These strategies set out a framework for improving access for those most in need and should include detailed action plans for tackling priority areas.

8.14 There are a number of different models of joint working ranging from information sharing and joint planning between separate agencies, to pooling of budgets and sharing of staff, or the establishment of care trusts. Experience shows that where there is a will to work jointly there is an ability to overcome barriers to improve outcomes. Where the will does not exist, formal structures are not enough. We do not want to impose solutions. Decisions about the best models to suit local circumstances should be made locally. **However, we are clear that doing nothing will not be an option**. We expect the local health and social care communities to work together with other voluntary and statutory agencies to take a community-wide approach to commissioning. This should include clarity about local leadership, accountability and partnership arrangements. Local partners can do this in a number of ways including, for example a virtual care trust or a partnership board of local agencies using the LSP as a framework, or they can explore other arrangements to meet these objectives.

8.15 The Government will support local partners in shifting the pattern of services towards cost-effective prevention, for example by building the evidence base of what works well and supporting the spread of best practice, aligning targets and performance frameworks, and developing mechanisms to promote a sustainable shift to a more effective pattern of preventative services across the whole system.

8.16 Other options could include:

- a mix of financial incentives tied to outcomes;
- use and development of the single assessment process, care programme approach and person-centred planning to develop joint pathways of care and integrated delivery networks;
- strengthening the duty for local councils and NHS commissioners to cooperate in commissioning services for adults;
- further use of shared workforce and IT initiatives which encourage joint working across health and social care boundaries;

- the enabling and encouragement of cross-commissioning arrangements for individual packages of care, eg community matrons and nurses commissioning home care, social workers commissioning equipment or other health-based interventions as part of a case-management role; and
- allowing councils to authorise other organisations to carry out a range of adult social services functions, including those involving the exercise of statutory discretion. The council would retain overall accountability and responsibility to ensure that their contracts with organisations carrying out functions conform to best practice, and include realistic but challenging performance measures and adequate monitoring arrangements.

Witham, Braintree and Halstead Care Trust was set up in 2002 and is responsible for the local health services for everyone living in the area and for social care services for local older people.

This means that there is now one organisation providing the services that older people used to receive from local NHS organisations, Essex County Council and Braintree District Council.

The trust can make sure that older people living locally can receive assessment and care management, home care support, sheltered housing, or residential care as part of an integrated package of care and is responsible for providing GP services, community hospital and nursing services, physiotherapy, and local general hospital services.

8.17 We anticipate that the DASS will play a key role in facilitating commissioning arrangements and that they will be monitored by the independent inspectorates, including the Commission for Social Care Inspection (CSCI), the Healthcare Commission and the Audit Commission. Outputs from the Care Services Efficiency Programme will also be available to support improved local commissioning.

Consultation questions

Your views are invited on the proposals set out in this chapter. In particular:

16. Do you support the proposal to develop a strategic commissioning framework?
17. Is the proposed shift to a preventative model of care the right approach?
18. What are your views on approaches to promoting and developing partnership working across agencies and effective models for so doing?

9. Service improvement and delivery

SUMMARY

This chapter recognises the challenges faced in improving the design and delivery of services, identifies support for service improvement, and gives some examples of innovative models of provision to stimulate wider debate.

9.1 Alongside the challenge to improve the strategic commissioning of services is the task of improving their design and delivery. This will mean radically different ways of working, redesign of job roles and reconfiguration of services. This will call for skills in leadership, communications and management of change of the highest order.

9.2 Service improvement is a crucial part of our vision. All too often the availability and quality of services have more to do with where people live than what they need or want. Direct payments, for example, are far more widely available in some areas than others, and inspections and joint reviews have found wide variations in the quality of services.[46] The Social Exclusion Unit (SEU) is running a number of projects which look at how mainstream services can better meet the needs of excluded people.[47] One of the projects on excluded older people particularly links to adult social care. Initial findings have highlighted the importance of low-level preventative services, the joining up of services, and the involvement of people using

services and local communities in service design creating choice and control. These key themes will be the focus of further work during 2005.

STRENGTHENING THE EVIDENCE BASE

9.3 Better services and improved outcomes are assisted by a firm knowledge base. The remit of social care is wide and, while there is a significant body of knowledge, in adult services in particular, the evidence has not always been used or developed. Dissemination of knowledge and good-quality research will help to support sound knowledge-based practice. This in turn will increase the confidence of workers in their ability to support genuine choice and independence. The Social Care Institute for Excellence (SCIE), which was set up in 2001, has made an important contribution to improved service delivery through making knowledge about good practice readily available.

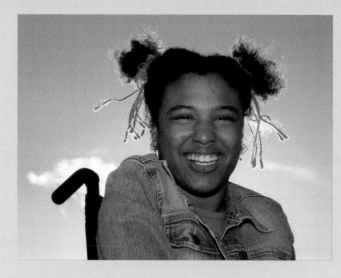

PULLING THINGS TOGETHER – AN IMPROVEMENT PARTNERSHIP FOR CARE SERVICES

9.4 We should not underestimate how challenging the concept of real choice might be. Once real choice is offered to those who use our services, for example through an individual budget, they will be empowered to reject the services that are currently on offer.

9.5 People who use services and carers must be involved in the design and shaping of the services they use. This might involve having a stronger voice in the way a care home or service is delivered, something that the Commission for Social Care Inspection (CSCI) is supporting and encouraging through its inspection and regulatory regime. It should also involve a much closer partnership between the people who use services and their families and carers, to identify needs, preferences and aspirations and to look at different ways in which these can be met. In local area agreement (LAA) pilot areas, for example, local authorities and the local strategic partnership are required to engage the voluntary and community sector fully in the design and delivery of their agreement with Government.

9.6 Much has already been achieved through the work of bodies such as the Local Government Association (LGA), the Association of Directors of Social Services (ADSS), the Improvement and Development Agency (IDeA), the Innovation Forum and local councils themselves to improve service delivery and performance. CSCI will continue to have a role, not only in inspections but also in service improvement, and we will encourage and foster all those who promote good practice and innovation and share learning.

9.7 There is a need for more direct support for local commissioners to shift the pattern of services and for local providers to consider how their services can be redesigned or refocused to provide the outcomes identified in *Independence, Well-being and Choice*. We are bringing together the following service improvement teams to create a Care Services Improvement Partnership:

- Health and Social Care Change Agent Team;
- Integrated Care Network;
- Integrating Community Equipment Services Team;
- National Child and Adolescent Mental Health Support Services;
- National Institute for Mental Health in England;
- Valuing People Support Team; and
- Change for Children Team.

9.8 We are keen to encourage local providers, including the voluntary and independent sectors, to work with people using services, their families and carers to develop new models of care that reflect our proposed outcomes. These will require effective partnerships between the social care and health sectors, between the statutory, voluntary and independent sectors, and between traditional social care providers and universal services. There is potential to unlock resources already within the system and to make more use of wider community capacity and voluntary sector support to create a more diverse range of services than is currently on offer, and in so doing better meet the needs of individuals.

9.9 Exciting models like *Supporting People*[48] (which helps people live independently in their own accommodation) are already challenging some of the assumptions we have made about the types of service best suited to some people. We offer an overview of some of these models to stimulate debate and discussion about innovative models of care to support our vision.

EXTRA CARE HOUSING

9.10 Extra care housing has been developed to give choice to very frail or disabled people whose care needs might traditionally have been met by residential care. It offers a model which allows people to live in their own homes with a range of facilities and support designed to meet their needs. Extra care housing can also form the basis of a range of intermediate care and outreach services, preventing older people from going into hospital or facilitating the discharge of those who have been in hospital.

St Catherine Court is a purpose-built development of 48 flats run by Hanover Housing Association in conjunction with Gloucestershire County Council Social Services and Gloucester City Council.

The scheme has a multicultural focus and is a real community. St Catherine Court includes six flats for younger people with disabilities, a big communal lounge, assisted bath and shower rooms, a guest room, hobbies room and other communal facilities, and care assistants on site 24 hours a day.

For the residents, moving to St Catherine Court has made a real difference to their lives. Janet and Colin moved to the scheme a few years ago. Colin had suffered two heart attacks and two strokes and could no longer cope with stairs or the garden at their old home. Two and a half years ago, Janet was diagnosed with cancer.

"We couldn't have been in a better place. We had all the support we needed. We can live independent lives with the security and support around when we need it. We couldn't have coped when Janet came out of hospital anywhere other than here. This is the ideal place for us to live and we have friends who say they need this now. There aren't enough places like this."

9.11 DH has initiated the Extra Care Housing Fund, which is providing £87 million in 2004–2006 to enable social services and their housing partners to provide new extra care housing. During the same period, the Housing Corporation funded £93 million. A further £60 million will be available for 2006–2008. DH has also supported the establishment of the Housing and Learning Improvement Network (Housing LIN), whose focus has been on establishing regional and local networks to disseminate good practice on the development and implementation of extra care housing strategies.

HOMESHARE

9.12 Homeshare is based on the simple idea of the exchange of housing for help. A householder offers housing to a home-sharer in exchange for an agreed level of support. This might include companionship, security, help with daily tasks, some financial support, or a combination of these. The success of such schemes will depend on proper assessment of home-sharers and local support for such arrangements.

Josie was referred to a Homeshare programme by a hospital after a stroke severely affected her behaviour. The hospital was keen to discharge her if home support could be arranged. She found a perfect match in Trevor, a young working man who needed accommodation and who handled her sometimes erratic ways with great diplomacy. Soon Josie came to admire Trevor and, keen to cook for him, regained her independence skills. Trevor stayed with her for three years by which time Josie was well enough to live alone again.[49]

ADULT PLACEMENT

9.13 Adult placement schemes help approved adult placement carers (ordinary people from the local community) to share their home or time with someone in need. Similar to fostering, but for adults, it is a highly flexible model and services can be tailored to meet the needs of a particular area or community group.

In Hackney, London, carers are being recruited from the orthodox Jewish community to provide short breaks for people with mental health needs and for older people with dementia who are also members of the orthodox community.

A scheme in north London is meeting the needs of the Black African and West Indian communities. It is managed by workers from those communities, and recruits carers through churches and mosques.

A scheme in Essex set up by the local primary care trust provides daytime support for frail older people. It has enabled people to stay in their own homes for longer and supports family carers to continue to care for their relatives.

In Lincolnshire, day care is provided for small groups of older people living in isolated rural communities, in the homes of locally recruited adult placement carers. Day-care programmes are tailored to the interests of the individuals in the group. The service is popular because it is responsive to the views of the participants and because people are no longer required to spend hours travelling to and from town-based day-care provision.

TECHNOLOGY-ENABLED SERVICES

9.14 Telecare has huge potential to support individuals to live at home, and to complement traditional care. It can give carers more personal freedom and more time to concentrate on the human aspects of care and support and will make a contribution to meeting potential shortfalls in the workforce.

Liverpool Telecare is a joint venture between Liverpool City Council and BT, set up as a way of alerting carers, relatives or neighbours to possible problems that people using services might have at home.

The home is fitted with a small number of sensors that monitor movements and activities and are able to detect such things as the person not getting up in the morning, abnormal usage of the fridge or cooker, or whether the person has not moved for a long time. People can be reminded to take their tablets, and if the automatic monitoring system detects that there might be a problem, a telephone call can be made to the person to check or to alert a carer.

9.15 Telecare is not only there to support frail older people. Technology has the capacity to transform the way we offer services and the support that is available to help people with dementia stay in their own homes. Technology provides a range of options to meet individual needs that can be adapted as those needs change. Early evidence from West Lothian[50] and Northamptonshire

indicates that investment in telecare services can have a significant impact on reducing the need for residential care, unlocking resources to be directed elsewhere in the system.

9.16 We are committed to transforming care services through the introduction of telecare, and the Government is currently planning to make £80 million available for two years from 2006 to local authorities to stimulate this transformation. We are currently working with a wide range of stakeholders to develop guidelines and strategies to support its introduction.

CONNECTED CARE CENTRES

9.17 The concept of connected care centres derives from *Meeting Complex Needs*.[51] Primarily a model for delivering health and social care support in the context of the wider community, connected care centres have the potential to meet the needs of those who have complex needs and live in deprived communities. This new model of delivery could enable local services to bridge the gap between health and social care and social inclusion strategies.

The key elements of a connected care centre are:
- a social care audit undertaken by members of the local community assisted by trained researchers to determine the size and shape of the centre;
- a service navigator with knowledge of all mainstream and specialist services who would work with the person using services to develop a sustained pathway of care;
- co-location of a variety of NHS, social care and community professionals;
- common assessment procedure;
- information sharing;
- shared training;
- single point of entry;
- round the clock support;
- managed transitions;
- continuing support; and
- individual budgets.

Hartlepool PCT, working with Turning Point, has agreement from the key local organisations, including the NHS, the wider local authority and community groups, for piloting this approach. A social care needs audit of the area will be undertaken, followed by the development of a connected care centre. There will also be an academic evaluation of the impact of this approach.

IMPROVED INFORMATION SHARING

9.18 We need to improve the early identification and response to people's needs through better assessment and information sharing between local councils and NHS services. The single assessment process for older people is a good model, which has been tested and implemented by more than four in five councils in England. It is based on a locally-agreed approach to overview assessment when people come into contact with health or social services, with specialist and comprehensive assessments undertaken for people with higher levels of need. This is a model that could usefully be extended to other groups in contact with statutory services.

Northern and Yorkshire Dementia Collaborative
Early identification of needs allows for an early response, as demonstrated by the Northern and Yorkshire Dementia Collaborative. In the Collaborative, people with dementia were identified much earlier than usual, resulting in the early mobilisation of support from social services, the NHS and the voluntary sector for the person and their family. This approach can be applied to the broad range of health and care needs as they emerge.

9.19 For people with complex needs, the challenge is not so much that of providing services, but ensuring a more coordinated response. As well as traditional sources of expertise in the care of people with complex needs from NHS secondary care specialists, new groups are emerging in social care and community and primary healthcare. These include social work case managers working in new ways, therapists working in intermediate care, occupational therapists, community pharmacists, advanced primary nurses, community matrons and general medical practitioners with special interests in the care of people with complex needs. Although many of these groups have a health background, people with complex needs require a coordinated health and social care response.

A pilot study is under way in three sites in England to determine how traditional and emerging groups of professionals can work together more effectively for people with complex needs. The study will help to identify the organisational and professional governance arrangements for the cross-agency, multi-professional working that will be needed to ensure that services for people with complex needs are designed around the needs of the person using services rather than those of the organisations and professionals who are involved in part of their care.

IMPROVING TRANSITION PLANNING

9.20 Young people with disabilities and other needs often start their adult lives hampered by poor transition planning between the child and adult parts of service provision and between agencies.

9.21 Good practice in transition planning does exist, but the Government has recognised that more needs to be done to ensure that all young people with disabilities have the chance to go on to adult lives where they can fulfil their potential. *Improving the Life Chances of Disabled People* recognises the importance of transition planning for the quality of life of people with disabilities and makes recommendations for improvement. We are proposing that the DASS should play a key role in ensuring that arrangements are in place to support individuals during the transition between different services, to ensure multi-agency coordination and a seamless pathway. Particular emphasis should be placed on maintaining a proper level of integration with adult social care services particularly in relation to learning disabilities, adult mental health and drug and alcohol services. Young people approaching the age of 18 should also be involved in planning the services that they will receive as adults in order to ensure that adult services are genuinely responsive to their needs.

Hamad has learning disabilities and lives with his family. Person-centred planning started in his final years at school. It made an immediate difference as it helped professionals and his family have a much better understanding of what was important to him. His health improved and he and his family became much happier with school. Planning was crucial to the transition, making sure that the services he was to use as an adult would work for him in vital areas such as personal care, diet and leisure interests. In Hamad's home town, these kinds of issues had sometimes led to people from South Asian communities being denied services. Person-centred planning and effective transition planning enabled everyone involved to focus on him as a unique individual, building commitment and pulling together to solve problems and remove obstacles. Hamad's mum says: "Planning has changed our lives. My son receives a service that guarantees meeting his personal and spiritual needs in the way which is important to him. We now have hopes and aspirations for his future. One in particular is to help him to buy his own house."

Consultation questions

Views are invited on the proposals set out in this chapter. In particular:

19. What help and support do local authorities and other social care providers need to work with people using services and carers to transform services?

20. Do you have innovative models of provision that support the outcomes of our vision?

10. Regulation and performance assessment

SUMMARY

This chapter recognises the importance of regulation and performance assessment as levers for challenge and change, and proposes that both should be modernised to reflect the outcomes of the vision.

10.1 Commissioners and providers of care services have the prime responsibility for ensuring that individual needs are met, but performance assessment, inspection and regulation are important levers to ensure that services are improved and appropriately focused on the right outcomes.

10.2 It is a generally accepted principle and one which we endorse that social care services need to have external inspection and regulation because:

- some people using those services are vulnerable to abuse and unable to speak out for themselves;
- it is difficult for existing and prospective users of services and their families to assess quality before choosing services, and difficult to change services if quality proves poor; and
- people are increasingly using their own resources to pay for social care and so do not have any support from their local council or the NHS.

The Care Standards Act 2000 signalled a strengthening of the regulatory regime. We now have:

- a single regulatory body for social care in England, the Commission for Social Care Inspection (CSCI), with additional powers to take an industry-wide view of social care, including the relationship between commissioning and provision of care services;
- a set of statutory regulations and underpinning national minimum standards (NMS), setting out for the first time the standards of care required across a wide spectrum including medication, staffing and the physical environment; and
- a General Social Care Council (GSCC) to regulate the social care workforce.

We have agreed in principle to merge CSCI and the Healthcare Commission into a single body by 2008, reflecting the increasing joint work between adult social care and health. The planned merger reflects shared objectives for the highest possible standards for everyone using social care and health services.

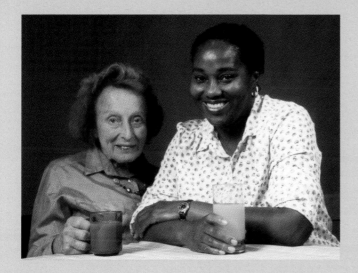

10.3 The development of this framework provides a firm foundation to encourage improvement in the quality of services and of the workforce.

10.4 Regulation based on the NMS is clearly having a positive impact in driving up the quality of registered services. Between 2002/03 and 2003/04, the proportion of care homes for older people which met each of the minimum standards rose from 26% to 48%, while care homes for younger adults meeting each minimum standard rose from 17% to 46%.

10.5 However, we are also told that the present regulatory regime could be improved. Many of the minimum standards focus on assessing prescriptive inputs rather than outcomes. The voices of people receiving social care services should be heard at all times, and the Government has recently accepted recommendations made by the Better Regulation Task Force on participation in social care regulation to ensure that this happens. In 2005, we will be publishing guidance to people using services and relevant organisations to clarify the position on payment for participation and ensure no one is deterred for financial reasons.

10.6 As services become more people-focused and more integrated across social care and health boundaries, existing inspection and performance assessment frameworks will play an important part in ensuring that our proposed outcomes and the vision are being delivered. The time is now right to modernise the approach to social care regulation, to be more proportionate, to reflect the aspirations of people using services properly, and to capture the quality and outcomes of the services provided. We have agreed with CSCI that it should take forward a programme of work to modernise regulation. CSCI has recently consulted on its proposals in *Inspecting for Better Lives*. In parallel we will be reviewing the relevant NMS and associated regulations.

PERFORMANCE MANAGEMENT

10.7 We know that our current system of performance measures does not match our proposed outcomes for social care and that there needs to be better alignment if they are to act as drivers for change. We are working within government on approaches to establishing possible well-being targets to underpin our policy on supporting people to maintain their independence. We will be working with CSCI to develop performance indicators that reflect the outcomes agreed as part of the consultation process on *Independence, Well-being and Choice*, and we expect that CSCI will use them as the basis for their performance assessment of local authorities.

10.8 Local strategic partnerships (LSPs) are also a major tool in helping to secure delivery by providing a framework for effective working across a number of agencies to achieve shared outcomes. In many local authorities partnership working between different agencies has long been a feature of service planning and delivery, but formalising LSPs can help to provide a clear focus and ensure clarity about the respective roles and responsibilities of different partners. LSPs will work with local agencies to secure agreements on outcomes and targets for specific cross-cutting issues and to monitor progress towards achieving them.

10.9 In summary, we plan to work to support delivery of the objectives we have set out through:

- aligning headline targets across relevant services with the objectives and outcomes we want;
- working with the inspectorates, local government and other stakeholders to develop performance measures and indicators that reflect and underpin the objectives, promoting continuous improvement; and
- ensuring that regulation and performance assessment and management systems for social care, the NHS and other services promote these objectives and local joint working towards them.

Consultation questions

Views are invited on the proposals set out in this chapter. In particular:

21. Do you have views on appropriate performance measures to encourage the implementation of the vision?
22. How can central government best enable LSPs develop and monitor progress on cross-cutting issues?

11. Building capacity: the workforce

SUMMARY

The workforce is critical to delivery of our vision. We want to support all staff to move to a model that supports and promotes the independence of people using services and carers. We are supporting initiatives in improving leadership and modernising the workforce and we will consider ways to improve local workforce planning.

THE WORKFORCE

11.1 People who use social care services say that the service is only as good as the person delivering it. They value social care practitioners who have a combination of the right human qualities as well as the necessary knowledge and skills. If we are to deliver our vision this means workers who are open, honest, warm, empathetic and respectful, who treat people using services with equity, are non-judgemental and challenge unfair discrimination.

11.2 We must generate a sustained change of culture to meet the challenges set by a more personalised approach to social care service delivery. Culture change of this form strengthens expectations on the workforce in terms of behaviours and values which are already set out in the General Social Care Council (GSCC) Code of Practice. At its core, it demands that we apply the principle of respect for all people using services, and act to end stigma and prejudicial attitudes. We need to develop a workforce that is reflective of the population it serves. Many of those who work in social care are already deeply committed to these ideals, but it is not true for all. More needs to be done to embed a shift towards supporting the wishes and human rights of people using services, and their family and community carers. Our approach must also be conscious of the reality of provision; well over half of the workforce is employed in the private sector.

SUPPORTING IMPROVED LEADERSHIP

11.3 If the change in focus and improved services to which we aspire are to be delivered, high-quality leadership will be essential. Leadership is about more than the contribution of senior managers and councillors. If real change is to come about in the way services are delivered, responding to the needs of those who use them, then we need people with vision and leadership skills at every level across the statutory, private and voluntary sectors.

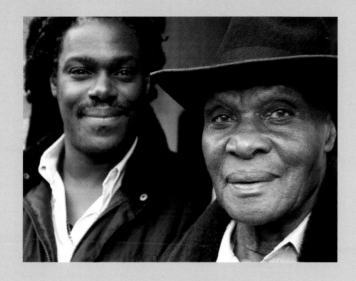

11.4 In October 2004, TOPSS England[52] launched a new national strategy for leadership and management,[53] which is widely supported by key partners. This new training and development strategy should make a significant contribution to strengthen management and leadership capacity in social care. It is now necessary to take this leadership strategy, and those being developed by other agencies' children's services, the NHS and local government and ensure that together they provide a powerful framework to improve leadership and management skills in social care and related public services.

11.5 For too long this workforce of over a million people has been undervalued. If we are to deliver the culture change that we seek, and deliver services that demonstrate the values we espouse, this needs to be addressed. Adult social care careers offer hugely challenging opportunities in a range of settings. We need to make social care an attractive career, in a way that embraces the purpose and fundamental worth of delivering people-centred care and draws in individuals from a wide variety of backgrounds. We also need to equip the workforce with the skills they will need to do the job.

11.6 Workforce development in adult social care should remain the responsibility of individual employers and Skills for Care, the employer-led sector skills council (SSC). We are asking for views on the direction that Government and other stakeholders should take to assist employers to recruit, retain and develop the people they need to deliver high-quality adult care services.

NEXT STEPS

11.7 Across the workforce agenda, we have already made some progress. The Modernising Social Services strategy has delivered increases in the size and skills of the workforce.

- Between 2001 and 2004, there has been a 45% increase in the number of students taking up a social care vocational course or degree programme.
- Access to financial support for every student since the Government introduced a £3,000 bursary in 2003.
- A register for social workers was opened in 2003 by the GSCC, to which 60,000 social workers have applied, and registration will be made a requirement for all social worker posts by April 2005.
- A programme of 28 pilot projects managed by TOPSS England to evaluate new types of worker will prove key to the delivery of our vision.

These and other signs of progress show that workforce change is having a key impact, but much remains to be done.

IMPROVING RECRUITMENT AND RETENTION

11.8 The current national vacancy rate across the social care workforce is 11%, which translates into around 110,000 unfilled posts. There has been an effective national recruitment campaign since 2001, but we still need to reduce vacancies across adult social care. We are committed to strengthening partnership with employers in the statutory, private and voluntary sectors and, in February 2005, TOPSS England became Skills for Care, a constituent council of the new UK SSC for social care, children and families. One of the key tasks of the new council will be to ensure improved workforce planning. Nationally, we are also supporting a new adult care network to bring together partner SSCs to help resolve common issues, support the further development of national recruitment and retention initiatives, and strengthen skills in interdisciplinary working. There is scope here both to address the problems in providing social care in remote rural areas, which are resistant to conventional service delivery due to inaccessibility, and also to reduce the problem of unemployment in some rural areas that contributes to the problems of social exclusion experienced by many people in the countryside.

11.9 In other areas of the public sector, where a culture of local workforce planning is more pervasive, workforce growth has exceeded that of the social care workforce. Taking forward effective workforce development at local, regional and national levels demands coherent and shared planning. Although there are excellent examples of shared workforce planning between private, public and voluntary sector providers, currently most planning is patchy and therefore does not support attempts to improve recruitment and retention. We are interested in your views about how better workforce planning could be achieved and better

integrated with the regional planning of SSCs and across to the health sector.

11.10 We also need to recognise that demographic changes will create pressures for a growing workforce if we continue to deliver care and support in traditional ways. It is important, therefore, that we look at developing and introducing different models of service delivery, such as telecare[54] which require a smaller workforce to deliver the support needed by an individual.

REWARDING STAFF

11.11 Although pay is not the only determinant of successful recruitment and retention, the experience of many employers suggests that reviewing pay and non-financial rewards which are valued by staff can lead to significant improvements in recruitment and retention. Some employers have discovered that a good part of the solution to retaining staff is for them to put 'whole-system' staff care policies in place. These can build on initiatives like Investors in People, or can learn from programmes like the NHS Improving Working Lives. Their aim is to establish practical support, personal development opportunities and workload management so that staff can look to their organisation as model employers who value their work and can offer them wider support to strike a better balance between their home and working lives. We propose to explore the value of such a nationally supported programme for social care workers.

11.12 In *Choosing Health*,[55] the Department of Health (DH) is committed to supporting NHS organisations in developing as healthier workplaces through development of a better evidence base to assess current practice, new guidance and dissemination of good practice, and initiatives to support leadership development. The Department is also initiating pilots to establish the effectiveness of promoting health in the workplace more generally in sectors outside the NHS.

TRAINING

11.13 TOPSS England has already started a fundamental review of the national training strategy, *Modernising the Social Care Workforce*, published in 2000. This review will examine the work undertaken since 2000 in setting new occupational standards and competencies for social care workers and in providing new frameworks for training. The intention is to launch a new national strategy for workforce development in 2006, which will provide a key opportunity to review the range of new skills and competencies that will be needed to implement our vision.

11.14 Much has been achieved in taking social work training to a new level over the last four years. There has been a significant increase in the number of students, a degree qualification has been established, and the GSCC is introducing a new framework for post-qualification learning. Despite these gains, there is more that can be done to support this profession at the heart of social care. The Government has established a group to consider further the development of social work jointly chaired by ministers from DH and the Department for Education and Skills (DfES). Social work will continue to have a key part to play in delivering better outcomes for people using services. Drawing on existing skills and the growing body of knowledge about what works well for people using services, social workers will be deployed in a variety of new settings and teams working alongside other professionals.

11.15 The workforce in general still has a poor level of training. It is estimated that no more than 25% of the workforce has a relevant qualification. This is not good enough, and it is important that the national minimum standards for training are met.

11.16 Some local authorities are providing training for carers. We would also like to see learning opportunities further extended to include volunteers, people using services and carers where possible. We know that training is good for those receiving care and it develops skills for carers both in supporting their current circumstances, and in providing a potential route into the workforce. Local authorities should consider whether this investment could in some circumstances prevent carer injury or breakdown.

WORKFORCE REGULATION

11.17 The GSCC opened the register for social workers in 2003. It will be an offence from April 2005 for people to call themselves a social worker unless they are registered with the GSCC. Work has also begun on registering the rest of the social care workforce. The GSCC has consulted on the next groups to register, and decisions will be made in summer 2005. Registration will assist in raising the status of the workforce and in setting standards of conduct and reducing risks to people using services.

FUNDING

11.18 Funding for significant further learning and workforce development is already in place. In addition to resources from other sources to support employers, such as Learning and Skills Councils, by 2005/06 the value of workforce development grants to employers from DH will have trebled since 2002 to around £225 million per annum.

Consultation questions

Views are invited on the proposals set out in these chapters. In particular:

23. Do you think the direction proposed for strengthening and developing skills in the workforce is right?
24. How can we improve and better integrate local workforce planning?
25. What actions are needed by Government and others to assist employers in recruiting, retaining and developing the workforce?

12. Community capacity building: working with the voluntary and community sector

SUMMARY

This chapter recognises the important role played by the voluntary and community sector (VCS) and sets out proposals for strengthening local engagement and building local capacity.

12.1 Support for a strong and vibrant VCS is an essential component of our vision and developing the well-being agenda. We want to encourage and support community capacity building at a local level. This will create opportunities for all citizens to contribute to society, to support people who may need assistance through volunteering, and to encourage the greater social inclusion of those who have traditionally been in receipt of help by giving them opportunities to contribute themselves.

12.2 The strategic commissioning role played by local government should provide an opportunity to engage more effectively with the VCS, in planning and delivering services. In the social care sector, commissioning as part of the wider pattern of local service delivery is well established and there is also some experience of developing local volunteering strategies. However, we would like to encourage local government to explore further the contribution of such strategies to deliver this vision. The development of a strong and long-term strategic relationship with VCS partners, through local contracts and local strategic partnerships

(LSPs) will support the development of better and more dynamic commissioning arrangements.

12.3 Those responsible for commissioning services should accept that it is legitimate for service providers in the VCS to factor in the relevant element of overhead costs into their cost estimates for services delivered under contract. Procurement contract performance measures should include customer satisfaction, as this is an area where VCS activity is likely to add value. Proposed contract sizes and contract lengths should allow service providers in the VCS to compete and the potential contribution of small organisations, particularly where there is an opportunity to develop services to meet the cultural needs of their community, should be considered. Commissioners should also ensure that monitoring, reporting and audit processes are proportionate and do not add unnecessary burdens to the VCS.

12.4 The VCS, volunteer organisations and user and family-led organisations are an integral part of the social care workforce, and their inclusion will add to the diverse capacity that is needed to

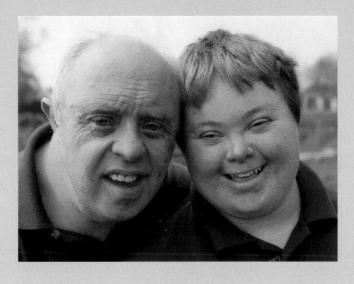

deliver our vision. The sector is able to play a vital role as an advocate in ensuring that people access the services they need. It can also have an important role in prevention, acting as an early warning system to avoid crises developing and in establishing clear referral channels with mainstream social services and the NHS.

Involving older people: a toolkit for the Active Elderly in South Holland

The Active Elderly project uses the skills and time of active older people to provide different types of support to people who are referred by a variety of statutory agencies. Services provided include help with paperwork, gardening, pet walking, or cooking a simple meal.

Funding for different aspects of the project has come from South Holland Primary Care Group (now the East Lincolnshire Primary Care Trust), Lincolnshire Social Services, the Countryside Agency, Help the Aged and Age Concern.

SUPPORTING LOCAL ENGAGEMENT

12.5 As a result of the Spending Review 2004, HM Treasury has been looking at specific areas of key public service delivery where there is potential for the VCS to add value. For the Department of Health (DH), the focus of its contribution was specifically on older people's services and, in particular, the implementation of the NSF for Older People standards on falls and stroke.

12.6 In collaboration with the Treasury and representatives from relevant VCS stakeholders, the Department explored where there might be most scope for the VCS to add value. While falls and stroke services were used as a focus for this work, the aim was to identify themes that could be applied more widely to other stakeholders and services.

12.7 This work concluded that there are already strong examples where the VCS has developed and is providing key elements of service provision to older people and that, given the right level of recognition and support, the VCS could and should be able to do more, not just for older people but for other groups as well.

12.8 There are some excellent examples of a holistic, person-centred approach, connection with local communities and understanding of the needs of people using services by the VCS which put it in a good position to work in partnership with the statutory agencies to deliver trusted, responsive and innovative services that people want.

12.9 By identifying and articulating what the VCS already does well, and encouraging it to participate in delivering our vision, public services can build the foundation for a more strategic engagement of the sector in service delivery and reform, and enable it to play a fuller role in the future.

12.10 At a local level, there needs to be more strategic engagement with the VCS by the relevant public sector commissioning authorities through the development of local compacts with VCS and participation in LSPs. To support local working, DH will:

- work with others to develop a cost-benefit analysis tool to inform local commissioning and investment decision making;
- spell out in more detail the overall role of the VCS in the context of National Service Frameworks to inform the Healthcare Commission and the Commission for Social Care Inspection's inspection criteria;
- develop Section 64[56] investment priorities so that they more closely reflect and support the delivery of strategic aims for health and social care service reform;
- support local area agreements, which mandate the full engagement of the VCS in agreeing shared outcomes and priorities; and
- take forward the strategic partnership agreement between DH, the NHS and the VCS, making partnership work for patients, carers and people using services through a new national strategic partnership forum to improve understanding of the benefits of VCS activity to health and social care delivery and overcome the barriers to achieving that.

12.11 In this way we expect to see the existing partnership between social care and the VCS growing and developing. We believe that a healthy voluntary sector and strong consumer/family organisations are good for the local community and provide opportunities to look at how the range of services or support can be extended to meet the needs of individuals. Not all services need to be provided by the statutory sector. Often volunteer services can develop interesting or novel approaches to meeting particular needs.

Helping Hands – a new social care partnership
Helping Hands is a demonstration project which started in December 2002.

Providing effective support for people in rural areas can be a particular challenge where public and private services are spread much more thinly and where remoteness and inaccessibility are often barriers. The Countryside Agency and Suffolk Social Care Services have developed the Community Support Co-operative to address some of the serious issues around home care and support service provision in rural Suffolk. The co-operative has piloted a new approach to service delivery where carers, support workers and customers are members of the not-for-profit organisation so that it can be tailored to the specific needs of the area.

12.12 We have already given examples in which the VCS has helped to develop innovative models of care, such as homeshare, and we believe that there is the opportunity in the sector to harness skills and creativity to contribute to the wider well-being agenda. One example of a creative solution to matching individual needs for support and the willingness of others to volunteer is in the use of time banks and we would like to see a greater exploration of their potential to contribute to local capacity building.

TIME BANKS
12.13 Time banks originated in the USA in the mid-80s, and are based on the concept of people using their time as money. Individuals build credits for time they put into voluntary activities in providing health or social care and other worthwhile work in their communities. Everybody's time is equally valued. Communities which are 'cash-poor, time-rich' are able to trade their time, providing each other with valuable services such as care for older people, family support or gardening. The time bank offers an opportunity to screen volunteers for suitability and reduces the risks involved in unregulated volunteering.

12.14 These schemes offer a means to reduce inequalities in health and encourage social inclusion because people become givers of time and they empower individuals with a feeling of self-worth. They provide communities with a means of trading services which they are denied by the conventional economy and they enable more support to be offered to the most socially disadvantaged people, who often experience poor health. They provide an opportunity for those who have traditionally been in receipt of care or services to offer something back to the community, increasing their sense of inclusion and having positive benefits for their own well-being.

Time banks are successfully attracting participants from socially excluded groups, including people in receipt of benefits, from low-income households, retired people and disabled people.

Time banks were felt to improve the quality of people's life and increase social interaction.

The values of time banking encourage people to develop practical visions for their neighbourhood. They know that others are there to help and support.[57]

About Waterloo Time Bank[58]

The Waterloo Time Bank was originally a pilot project set up in St John the Evangelist Church in 2002.

It aims to involve local people and organisations in creating informal systems of neighbours helping neighbours. This concept encourages a spirit of equality by creating opportunities for socially excluded people to be valued as productive members of society with their own unique contribution.

Waterloo is divided by transport and local government boundaries but it is a diverse and interesting community. There is a wide range of different cultures and, during the day, workers, university students and students from the local English-language schools frequent the area. The Waterloo Time Bank has proved popular with English-language students who exchange their skills for conversational English. Within Waterloo there are several complexes of sheltered housing. Chaplin Close sheltered housing has benefited from the Waterloo Time Bank by having a garden designed and maintained by time bank members.

Consultation question

Views are invited on the proposals set out in this chapter. In particular:

26. How can we strengthen the links with the VCS and increase community capacity?

13. Conclusion and next steps: how you can contribute

13.1 We would like to thank you for taking the time to read *Independence, Well-being and Choice*. In summary, we have talked about:

- how we can offer more control, more choice and high-quality support for those who use care services;
- how we can harness the capacity of the whole community so that everyone has access to the full range of universal services and an opportunity to play a full part in society; and
- how we can improve the skills and status of the workforce to deliver the vision.

13.2 Our key proposals to deliver this vision include:

- wider use of direct payments and individual budgets to stimulate the development of modern services delivered in the way people want;
- greater focus on preventative services to allow for early targeted interventions and a harnessing of the local authority well-being agenda to ensure greater social inclusion and improved quality of life;

- a strong strategic and leadership role for local government, working in partnership with other agencies, particularly the NHS, to ensure a wide range of effective and well-targeted provision, which meets the needs of our diverse communities; and
- encouraging the development of new and exciting models of service delivery and harnessing technology to deliver the right outcomes for adult social care.

13.3 The ideas we have put forward in *Independence, Well-being and Choice* are to encourage and stimulate discussion about the future direction for adult social care. We would now like to hear your views on our proposals so that together we can move forward towards implementing a shared vision and create a social care environment which is right for the 21st century.

THE CONSULTATION PROCESS

13.4 At the end of each chapter are a list of questions on which we would like your views. But we are also interested to hear from you about any aspect of *Independence, Well-being and Choice* and, in particular, whether you think that the vision we have set out is the right one.

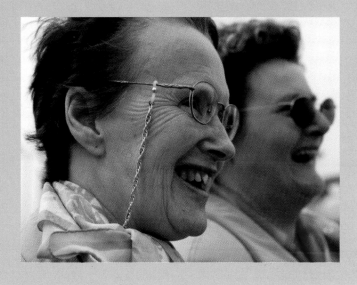

13.5 We also welcome any comments you have on the Regulatory Impact Assessment (RIA) of *Independence, Well-being and Choice* and on the separate consultation on guidance on the role of the Director of Adult Social Services, both of which can be found on the internet at www.dh.gov.uk/socialcare. Contributions on changing the name of direct payments and extending their scope can be found in appendices C and D.

13.6 To take part in these consultations, response forms can be completed online or downloaded from www.dh.gov.uk/socialcare. Alternatively you may write in or e-mail. Completed questionnaires and other responses should be sent to the address shown below by 28 July 2005.

By post:

Adult Social Care Green Paper
Consultation Unit
Department of Health
Wellington House
133–155 Waterloo Road
London
SE1 5UG

By e-mail: adultsocialcare@dh.gsi.gov.uk

13.7 The information that you send to us may need to be passed to colleagues within the Department of Health and other government departments and/or published in a summary of responses to this consultation. We will assume that you are content for us to do this and if you are replying by e-mail, that your consent overrides any confidentiality disclaimer that is generated by your organisation's IT system, unless you specifically include a request to the contrary in the main text of your submission to us. Please ensure that if you want your name or response to be kept confidential, you state this clearly in your response. (Confidential responses will be included in any statistical summary of numbers of comments received and views expressed.)

13.8 All written, public consultations must follow the Cabinet Office Code of Practice on Consultation. The full text of the code of practice is on the Cabinet Office website at www.cabinetoffice.gov.uk/regulation/consultation/code.asp.

The code contains six criteria for us to follow:

- Consult widely throughout the process, allowing a minimum of 12 weeks for written consultation at least once during the development of the policy.

- Be clear about what your proposals are, who may be affected, what questions are being asked and the timescale for responses.
- Ensure that your consultation is clear, concise and widely accessible.
- Give feedback regarding the responses received and how the consultation process influenced the policy.
- Monitor your department's effectiveness at consultation, including with a designated consultation coordinator.
- Ensure your consultation follows better regulation best practice, including carrying out a Regulatory Impact Assessment (RIA) if appropriate.

13.9 The code also requires us to reproduce these criteria in consultation documents, explain any departure from the code and confirm that all other criteria are followed. Criterion 3 of the code requires us to 'invite respondents to comment on the extent to which the criteria have been adhered to and to suggest ways of further improving the consultation process'. We must also 'explicitly state who to contact if respondents have comments or complaints about the consultation process'. For Department of Health consultations, comments or complaints should be directed to:

Steve Wells
Consultations Coordinator
Department of Health
Skipton House
80 London Road
London SE1 6LH

By e-mail: steve.wells@dh.gsi.gov.uk

APPENDICES

Appendix A
Acknowledgements

The ideas in this Green Paper have been developed through listening to a wide range of stakeholders during the spring, summer and autumn of 2004.

We are particularly indebted to the Social Care Institute for Excellence (SCIE) which undertook a consultation on the 'vision for social care' on our behalf with people who use and work in social care services. The results of this consultation are available at www.scie.org.uk.

Our thanks go to the following organisations who formally contributed to the discussions either at meetings with officials or ministers or in writing:

Abbeyfield Society

Action on Elder Abuse

Action with Communities in Rural England

Age Concern England

Alzheimer's Society

Anchor Trust

Association for Real Change

Association of Directors of Social Services

Beth Johnson Foundation

Care and Repair England

Carers UK

Charles Leadbeater, DEMOS

Commission for Social Care Inspection

Counsel and Care

CRISIS

Crossroads 'Caring for Carers'

Disabled Living Foundation

Disabled Parents Network

Ethnic Minority Foundation

Foundation for People with Learning Disabilities

General Social Care Council

Help the Aged

Improvement and Development Agency

Institute for Public Policy Research

Leonard Cheshire

Local Government Association

Long-term Medical Conditions Alliance

Mencap

Mind

Motor Neurone Disease Association

MS Society

National Association of Adult Placement Services

National Pensioners Convention

Parkinson's Disease Society

Princess Royal Trust for Carers

RADAR

Royal National Institute of the Blind

Royal National Institute for Deaf People

Sane

SCOPE

Social Policy Research Unit at York University

Stroke Association

The Mental Health Foundation

The National Council on Independent Living

The Tavistock Institute

Turning Point

Values in Action

Thanks also go to all those individuals and other organisations who took the trouble to write to the Department of Health by e-mail directly through the mailbox adultsocialcare@dh.gsi.gov.uk.

Appendix B

Glossary

Access to Work (AtW)
This is available to help overcome the problems resulting from disability. As well as giving advice and information to disabled people and employers, Jobcentre Plus pays a grant, through AtW, towards any extra employment costs that result from a person's disability.

Association of Directors of Social Services (ADSS)
A membership organisation which represents all the directors of social services in England, Wales and Northern Ireland.

Attendance Allowance (AA)
A non means-tested, non-contributory benefit paid as a contribution towards the extra costs associated with disability where a person becomes disabled or benefit is claimed after the age of 65. It is paid at two rates, depending on the level of need.

Audit Commission (AC)
An independent public body responsible for ensuring that public money is spent economically, efficiently and effectively in the areas of local government, housing, health, criminal justice and fire and rescue services.

Better Regulation Task Force (BRTF)
An independent body that advises government on action to ensure that regulation and its enforcement accord with five principles of good regulation.

Building community capacity
Development work that strengthens the ability of communities and community organisations to build local skills, structures, participation and solutions.

Care Direct
Care Direct comprised six pilots in the South West which tested models for working in partnership. The lessons learnt from the pilots are feeding into the developments of Link-Age.

Care programme approach (CPA)
The process which mental health service providers use to coordinate the care for people who have mental health problems.

Care Services Efficiency Delivery Programme
Established by the Department of Health to support implementation of the recommendations of Sir Peter Gershon's independent review of public sector efficiency.

Care trusts
Organisations that work in both health and social care. They may carry out a range of services, including social care, mental health services or primary care services.

Commission for Social Care Inspection (CSCI)
The single, independent inspectorate for all social care services in England.

Community matrons

A new role for nurses, announced in January 2005, which will enable them to give one-to-one support to patients with long-term conditions.

Direct Payment

State pensions and benefits paid directly into an individual's bank or other account.

Direct payments

Financial resources given to people so that they can organise and pay for the services that they need, rather than use the services that the council offers.

Disability Living Allowance (DLA)

A social security benefit which may be paid to people under 65 who have a long-term health problem, mental or physical, that affects their everyday activities.

Fair Access to Care Services (FACS)

Guidance issued by the Department of Health to councils and care trusts about fair charging policies for home care and other non-residential care, and advice about eligibility criteria for adult social care.

Family Fund

The Family Fund is an independent organisation registered as a charity. The purpose of the Fund is to ease the stress on families in the UK who care for severely disabled/seriously ill children aged 15 and under, by providing grants related to the care of the child.

General Social Care Council (GSCC)

The social care workforce regulator. It registers social care workers and regulates their conduct and training.

Healthcare Commission

This promotes improvement in the quality of healthcare in England and Wales. In England this includes regulation of the independent healthcare sector.

Improvement and Development Agency (IDeA)

This exists to stimulate and support continual and self-sustaining improvement and development within local government.

Independent Living Fund

The Independent Living Funds were set up as a national resource dedicated to the financial support of disabled people to enable them to choose to live in the community rather than in residential care.

Innovation Forum

This was created to promote dialogue between central and local government and its partners, on new ways of working to deliver better services to local communities.

Learning and Skills Council (LSC)

This exists to improve the skills of England's young people and adults to make sure we have a workforce that is of a world-class standard.

Local area agreement (LAA)

This provides a single framework through which government departments can allocate additional funding to a local authority and its partners.

Local Government Association (LGA)

This represents the local authorities of England and Wales to promote better local government.

Local Public Service Agreement (LPSA)

An agreement between a local authority and Government with targets to improve services in return for extra funding.

Local strategic partnership (LSP)

The LSP brings agencies and others together in a way which focuses and commits its members to improving the quality of life and governance in a particular area.

Long-term conditions

Those conditions that cannot, at present, be cured but can be controlled by medication and other therapies. They include diabetes, asthma, and arthritis.

Modernising Social Services
A White Paper issued in 1998 setting out a strategy for promoting independence, improving protection and raising standards.

National minimum standards (NMS)
NMS are set by the Department of Health for a range of services, including care homes, domiciliary care agencies and adult placement schemes. The CSCI must consider the NMS in assessing social care providers' compliance with statutory regulations.

National Service Frameworks (NSFs)
Long-term strategies for improving specific areas of care. There is a rolling programme, which includes older people and long-term conditions.

NHS Improvement Plan
This sets out the Government objective of providing better support and improving the quality of life for people with illnesses or medical conditions that they will have for the rest of their lives, by providing high-quality personal care.

Person-centred planning (PCP)
This is a process of life planning for individuals based on the principles of inclusion and the social model of disability.

Prime Minister's Strategy Unit
This unit provides the Prime Minister and government departments with a capacity to analyse major policy issues and design strategic solutions.

Regional Housing Boards (RHBs)
These have specific responsibility in England for the preparation of a regional housing strategy to achieve sustainable communities.

Section 64
The Section 64 General Scheme grants are made to voluntary organisations in England whose activities support the Department of Health's policy priorities.

Single assessment process (SAP)
This aims to make sure older people's care needs are assessed thoroughly and accurately, but without procedures being needlessly duplicated by different agencies.

Social Care Institute for Excellence (SCIE)
Using knowledge gathered from diverse sources, SCIE develops and promotes knowledge about good practice to support those working in social care and empower service users.

Social exclusion
The process that can take place when people or areas suffer from a combination of linked problems such as unemployment, poor skills, low incomes, poor housing, high-crime environments, bad health and family breakdown.

Social Exclusion Unit (SEU)
Part of the Office of the Deputy Prime Minister, it works to create prosperous, inclusive and sustainable communities for the 21st century by running projects to tackle specific issues of social exclusion.

Supporting People
A working partnership of local government, service users and support agencies to provide high-quality and strategically planned housing-related services.

Universal services
Services provided to the whole community. These can include education and health, libraries, leisure facilities and transport.

Voluntary and community sector (VCS)
Over half a million voluntary and community groups in the UK, ranging from small community groups to large national or international organisations.

Appendix C

Extending the scope of direct payments

Introduction

Direct payments were first introduced in 1997 for working age adults and, over time, have been opened up to older people in 2000, and in 2001 to parents of disabled children and carers. Regulations that came into force on 8 April 2003 put a duty on councils to make direct payments to individuals who consent to and are able to manage, with or without assistance.

Our aim, in promoting direct payments, is to increase individuals' independence and choice by giving them control over the way the services they receive are delivered. We recognise that most people prefer to live independently in their own homes and direct payments are a good way to support this.

Policy intention of extending direct payments

The intention is to extend the scope of direct payments payable to adults under the Health and Social Care Act 2001 to those currently excluded from having a direct payment, either because they cannot consent to a direct payment or cannot manage, even with assistance. This will give them the equivalent benefits of flexibility and a personalised service.

Who should have a direct payment?

Currently, for an individual to receive a direct payment, they must consent to it, and be able to manage the payment on their own or with whatever assistance is available to them. It is not our intention that direct payments should be made to people who do not want to have them.

The intention is to extend the benefits of direct payments to those who cannot consent to a direct payment and to those who lack the ability to manage, where this is in their best interest and to enable a more person-centred approach to their care.

However, when deciding whether someone lacks capacity to consent or to manage payments, it will be necessary to work within the Mental Capacity Bill which, subject to parliamentary approval, is expected to be implemented in 2007. This requires us to assume that a person has capacity unless it is established that they lack it. Under the Bill, people must be empowered to make as many decisions as possible for themselves. A council will therefore have to be satisfied that someone lacks capacity to consent or to manage payments, even with assistance, before these additional arrangements are considered. We would expect this assessment to be done by a qualified social worker or care manager when either reviewing or assessing an individual's need for services.

Where an individual may benefit from the flexibility and person-centred nature of a direct payment, but is not able to consent to have one, or cannot manage, even with assistance, we intend that councils should consider nominating an agent to manage the direct payment on that individual's behalf. In accordance with the Mental Capacity Bill, local councils will need to support individuals to make their own decisions wherever possible. In those situations where it is not possible for the individual to make the decision, they should involve the individual as much as is possible, even if they do not make the final decision.

Direct payments nominated to an agent will be considered in circumstances where it is clear that a payment in lieu of services would provide the most effective means for securing services appropriate to the needs of the person requiring services. They should only be offered where the council is satisfied that they will be in the best interests of the individual and are not against their stated preferences. Councils will only make a direct payment in this way where they are satisfied that it will meet the assessed need of the individual and will also need to be satisfied that the needs, desires and preferences of the person needing support are central to the way in which the direct payment will be used.

It is expected that this proposal will help to extend the use of payments in lieu of services to many more people, including:

- young disabled people whose parents have managed a direct payment on their behalf, and whose payments may have to stop when they reach the age of 18;
- people with dementia where the use of direct payments is not set out in a power of attorney agreement; and
- people with more profound learning disabilities.

Direct payments can already be made to parents of disabled children in this way. We are not proposing any changes to the way this operates.

We think that it is unlikely that there will be any circumstances in which a carer might benefit from a direct payment, but cannot either consent to a direct payment, or manage even with assistance, but would welcome views.

There are a very small group of people who are currently excluded under regulations, because they are subject to restrictions under mental health legislation (or certain related criminal justice measures).

Do you think we should now review these exclusions?

Do you think that extending direct payments should initially be a power for local councils, or a duty?

We expect this to be a duty on local councils, as for all direct payments.

Who should a direct payment be paid to, if not the individual?
How the council decides who should manage the payment once the local authority has taken a decision that someone does not have the capacity to consent to a direct payment, or to manage one even with assistance, will be the crucial element. In this case an 'agent' should be nominated, whether this is a carer or family member, a trust arrangement, or another arrangement that is suited to the individual's needs and circumstances. Local councils will want to consider carefully who the agent should be in each individual case and be confident that they will work in the best interests of the individual, that there are no grounds for concerns about abuse with appropriate checks having been made and that they will be able to manage the payment themselves, with assistance. In making this decision, councils and agents will need to operate

within the framework of the Mental Capacity Bill. Under the Bill, all decisions must be made in the best interests of the person who lacks capacity. The Bill will be accompanied by a code of practice that gives details on how to determine what is in someone's best interests. Guidance will need to be provided to agents to enable them to comply with this. Models such as the In Control project will help local councils make these decisions.

Councils will need to ensure that people have access to appropriate advice and support so that they understand the responsibilities involved before agreeing to take on the management of a direct payment.

As with direct payments, people taking on management of a direct payment for someone else are taking on an agreement with the council that they will meet the needs which have been identified through an assessment to an adequate standard.

Councils should focus on building supportive networks which can help to ensure the person requiring support remains at the centre of the arrangements made with the payment and that a well-balanced and informed understanding of the individual's preferences is used to provide active feedback to monitor and adjust the package to best suit the individual's needs and desires.

Before agreeing to an agent taking on the management of a direct payment, the council will be satisfied that there is no conflict of interest between the person requiring services and the agent.

One restriction that we think should be imposed is that the agent should not generally be able to pay themselves to provide the service. This is to ensure that the person managing the payment is independent of the provision of the service. However, there may be occasions when the most appropriate agent and the person best placed to deliver the care may be the same person. Local councils will need to look at each individual case, and put in place mechanisms to manage this discussion.

What should a direct payment be used for?

We intend that this extension of the direct payments legislation should apply to the same services as those under the existing direct payments legislation. Not all social care services are included in the direct payments legislation, although a great many of the services for which local councils are responsible are. The legislation applies to:

- a community care service within the meaning of Section 46 of the National Health Service and Community Care Act 1990; or
- a service under Section 2 of the Carers and Disabled Children Act 2000; or
- a service which local councils may provide under Section 17 of the Children Act 1989 (provision of services for children in need, their families and others).

As stated above, we are not proposing to change the legislation as it relates to children or carers, but to all other services covered under this legislation.

How will the service be provided?

Local councils will agree how the care plan will be delivered with the individual's agent and then monitor this through the normal care management review process. This process applies to an individual receiving a service directly from the council or via a direct payment. Councils will need to be satisfied that an individual's identified care needs are being met in every case, and the arrangements to do so should be the same for everyone, regardless of how the service is provided. Councils also regularly monitor how money is spent by direct payment recipients. The same arrangements should continue as we widen the scope of direct payments.

The agent will take on all the responsibilities that direct payment recipients currently hold, which can include becoming an employer, buying services from an agency, etc. Agents would also need to act in accordance with the Mental Capacity Bill, when making a decision about the individual receiving the service. That is, they will need to allow the person lacking capacity to make as many decisions for themselves as possible and they must act in their best interests. The Bill, and accompanying code of practice, set out details on how to make an objective assessment of what is in someone's best interests.

Councils will need to ensure that all people using direct payments are treated equitably. Thus, for example, people receiving a direct payment on someone else's behalf will have the same responsibilities for ensuring care is delivered to an adequate standard, and that all legal requirements are met. The recording requirements placed on agents will be the same as if the person were receiving direct payments themselves, to show evidence of how the money has been spent in order to deliver care. Equally, the way in which charges are dealt with should be the same for all users of direct payments, as with those receiving a service directly provided by the council. Councils will want work in partnership with the agent taking on the management of a direct payment to help them make arrangements which protect and promote the interests of the person needing services. Most people wishing to use a direct payment will be willing and able to do this, but councils should only arrange a direct payment in this way where they are satisfied that this is the case.

Councils should aim to ensure that the preferences and choices of the person requiring services are reflected in the make-up of services purchased with the direct payment. Feedback from the individual using the services purchased should be considered central to monitoring the success of the arrangements and considering any adjustments.

Support should be given to carers or others who are willing to take on this role, much in the same way as direct payment recipients currently receive. For direct payments this has proved essential to the successful operation of a direct payment, and those areas with the most people on direct payments are those where a good support service is in place. Agents may need

particular types of support which differ from those needed by people managing their own direct payments. Councils will want to ensure that this is reflected in their commissioning arrangements with providers of local support schemes.

In some cases, establishing formal trust arrangements may be a helpful way of ensuring that services are managed appropriately on behalf of users and that there is a range of voices which can give a well-rounded consideration to whether the users' best interests are being met. In other cases the same aims can be achieved with a less formal arrangement such as utilising a circle of support. Support services and local advocacy services may be well placed to participate in the circle of support/trust arrangement for managing the payment. This should be a decision taken with the full involvement of all the individuals concerned. We would not expect councils to make a blanket decision about how arrangements will work, but respond to the needs of each individual.

We think the existing restrictions on employing close relatives with a direct payment should be applied.

> What do you think about the proposal to extend direct payments via an agent to groups currently excluded, namely those unable to give consent or unable to manage a payment, even with assistance?

How to respond
Details of how to respond to this consultation can be found in paragraph 13.6 of the main document.

What will happen next?
A summary of responses, including the next steps, will be published on www.dh.gov.uk and paper copies will be available on request.

Appendix D

Changing the name of direct payments

Introduction

This appendix sets out the Department of Health's (DH's) plans to change the name of direct payments. We will also be working with the Department for Education and Skills (DfES) as direct payments are not only made to disabled people aged 16 or over, but also to people with parental responsibility for disabled children, and to young people aged 16 and 17.

Background

From 1999, the Department for Work and Pensions (DWP) has been using the term 'Direct Payment' to describe how individuals receive their benefit or pension directly into a bank account. This has caused confusion with the direct payments for people using local councils' services, which give cash payments to people to buy their own care.

Direct payments for social care

Direct payments in this context mean payments to individuals who have been assessed as needing services, to arrange their own care.

Direct payments for adults of working age were introduced in April 1997, through the Community Care (Direct Payments) Act 1996. They were extended to older disabled people in 2000. Since April 2001 (Carers and Disabled Children Act 2000) direct payments have been available

to carers, parents of disabled children and 16 and 17 year olds.

The Health and Social Care Act 2001 paved the way for a variety of changes to the way in which direct payments schemes operate, and regulations came into force in April 2003 that require councils to make direct payments to people using community care services who can choose to have them.

Direct Payment to pay benefits and pensions

DWP has a target of paying 85% of their customers directly into their accounts by 2005. This actually means that over a two-year period (which runs up to April 2005), they will be contacting over 13 million people and asking them to change how they are paid their money. This has been a huge task, and finding a suitable way to get this message across was important.

Independent customer research showed that the name and style of information enables customers to quickly and clearly understand the changes. DWP continually track the effectiveness of their information campaign and so far it is very successful in communicating the change to payment into an account.

The proposals

We have heard on many occasions the confusion the term 'direct payment' has caused to both providers and users of the service. We understand those concerns and therefore want to change the name of direct payments, not only to prevent them being confused with a direct payment for pensions or benefits, but also to take the opportunity to find a name that suits the purpose of local council direct payments and their aims. We need your help and suggestions to do this.

We have some initial thoughts, and would like to know your views about which describes more accurately what a direct payment is for, and will be the most easy for people to use and understand. We have already ruled out 'independent living payments' as this will only cause further confusion with the Independent Living Fund.

Suggestions for name change

Which of these do you think is the most appropriate? Are there any others?
- direct services payments
- individual service payments
- individualised funding
- personal budget

How will the change work?

Direct payments were created by the Community Care (Direct Payments) Act 1996, and are now made under the Health and Social Care Act 2001. This means that the name is defined in legislation.

DH will seek a legislative opportunity to change the name of direct payments. However, we will use the new name officially in all references to direct payments from April 2006.

Councils will not be under an obligation to make this change. However, the national message will be changing, and given that DH will seek to change the law at the earliest opportunity they will be well advised to make the change at the same time.

This change will also affect people living in Wales, as the legislative base for direct payments in Wales is the same, the Community Care (Direct Payments) Act 1996. The Welsh Assembly is not considering a name change at this stage, but may undertake their own consultation in the future.

Timescale for change

We appreciate that it will take time for a new name to be introduced. Councils and voluntary organisations will need to help people using direct payments get used to a new name, and to produce new information materials.

DH and DfES will ensure that any reprints or new publications and/or guidance will reflect the new name change.

We think that councils will need to have the new name in force by April 2006, but we need to hear from you if this is reasonable.

When do you think the change should be introduced?

How to respond

Details of how to respond to this consultation can be found in paragraph 13.6 of the main document.

What will happen next?

A summary of responses, including the next steps, will be published on www.dh.gov.uk and paper copies will be available on request.

We may need, at a later stage, to amend the direct payments legislation.

We will reissue our guidance and update all our publications with the new name as they go out of print. This is likely to be by April 2006.

References

1   The policies and proposals it contains apply to England only.

2   A Regulatory Impact Assessment (RIA) to accompany the proposals in this paper has been prepared and is available on the Department of Health website at www.dh.gov.uk/socialcare. In addition to commenting on the proposals in this paper, you may wish to comment on the contents of the RIA which will be revised during the course of the consultation to take account of up-to-date information.

3   Community Care (Direct Payments) Act 1996.

4   Prime Minister's Strategy Unit (2005) *Improving the Life Chances of Disabled People*, Recommendation 4.5: Piloting Individualised Budgets.

5   Office for National Statistics (2001) *Living in Britain, General Household Survey 2001,* HMSO: London.

6   Countryside Agency and NCH (2000) *Challenging the Rural Idyll.* Countryside Agency: London.

7   Royal Commission on Long-term Care for the Elderly, 1999.

8   Government Actuary, 2004.

9   Department for Environment, Food and Rural Affairs (2004) *Social and economic change and diversity in rural England,* Defra: London.

10 University of Lancaster Institute for Health Research for the Department of Health Learning Disability Task Force.

11 Audit Commission (2000) *Forget-me-not: Mental health services for older people,* Audit Commission: London.

12 Association of the British Pharmaceutical Industry estimates.

13 Collishaw, S, Maughan, B, Goodman, R and Pickles, A (2004) *Time Trends in Adolescent Health,* Nuffield Foundation: London.

14 Commission for Social Care Inspection findings.

15 Commission for Social Care Inspection (2004) *A Vision for Adult Care – Feedback from physically and sensory disabled people in local service inspection,* CSCI: London.

16 Department of Health (2000) *No Secrets: Guidance on developing and implementing multi-agency policies and procedures to protect vulnerable adults from abuse,* DH: London.

17 Sir Michael Bichard (2004) *The Bichard Inquiry Report,* TSO: London.

18 *Improving the Life Chances of Disabled People,* Recommendation 4.7.

19 *Improving the Life Chances of Disabled People.*

20 Department of Health (2001) *National Service Framework for Older People.* Single assessment process. DH: London.

21 Department of Health (1990) *Care Programme Approach HC(90)23/LASSL(90)11,* DH: London.

22 Department of Health (2001) *Valuing People: A New Strategy for Learning Disability for the 21st Century,* DH: London.

23 Department of Health (2005) *Supporting People with Long-term Conditions: An NHS model to support local innovation and integration,* DH: London.

24 Department of Health (2004) *NHS Improvement Plan: Putting people at the heart of public services,* DH: London.

25 Community Care (Direct Payments) Act 1996.

26 Joseph Rowntree Foundation (2004) *Making direct payments work for older people,* www.jrf.org.uk/knowledge/findings/socialcare/234.asp.

27 Commission for Social Care Inspection data, September 2003.

28 In Control, sponsored by Mencap. www.selfdirectedsupport.org

29 Clark, H, Gough, H and Macfarlane, A (2004) *'It pays dividends': Direct payments and older people*, The Policy Press and DH: London.

30 *Improving the Life Chances of Disabled People*, Recommendation 4.5: Piloting Individualised Budgets.

31 Department of Health (2004) *Choosing Health: Making healthier choices easier*, DH: London.

32 Section 31: Partnership arrangements.

33 Section 2: Economic, social and environmental well-being powers.

34 Sir Peter Gershon (2004) *Gershon Review: Releasing Resources for the Frontline: Independent Review of Public Sector Efficiency*, HM Treasury: London.

35 Zarb, G and Nadash, P (1994) *Cashing in on Independence: Comparing the costs and benefits of cash and services.*

36 *Older People: Independence and Well-Being*, Audit Commission, 2004.

37 *Fair Access to Care Services: Guidance on eligibility criteria for adult social care*, Department of Health Circular LAC(2002)13

38 Any new obligations on local government should be matched by appropriate funding from the responsible department.

39 Office of the Deputy Prime Minister (2003) *Sustainable Communities: Building for the Future*, ODPM: London.

40 Clark, H, Dyer, S and Horwood, J (1998) *That little bit of help: the high value of low-level preventative services for older people*, The Policy Press: London.

41 Department of Health (2000) *Shaping the future NHS: long-term planning for hospitals and related services consultation document on the findings of the national beds inquiry*, DH: London.

42 www.dh.gov.uk/PolicyAndGuidance/HealthAndSocial CareTopics/OlderPeoplesServices/fs/en.

43 Office of the Deputy Prime Minister (2004) *The Future of Local Government: Developing a 10-year vision*, ODPM: London.

44 Social Exclusion Unit (2001) *A New Commitment to Neighbourhood Renewal: A National Strategy Action Plan*, SEU: London.

45 *The Future of Local Government.*

46 *All Our Lives: Social Care in England 2002–3*, Audit Commission, Social Services Inspectorate and National Care Standards Commission.

47 Social Exclusion Unit (2004) *Young Adults with Troubled Lives, Excluded Older People, Frequent Movers, Disadvantaged Adults*, www.socialexclusion.gov.uk.

48 Office of the Deputy Prime Minister (2003) *Supporting People*, ODPM: London.

49 Homeshare International, www.homeshare.org.

50 *Opening Doors for Older People*, West Lothian Council.

51 Rankin, J and Regan, S (2004) *Meeting Complex Needs: The Future of Social Care*, Institute for Public Policy Research and Turning Point: London.

52 Training Organisation for the Personal Social Services (TOPSS) England.

53 *Leadership and Management: a strategy for the social care workforce*, TOPSS England, October 2004.

54 See chapter 9, Technology-enabled services.

55 *Choosing Health.*

56 Grants introduced in 1968 to help voluntary organisations whose work supports the Government's health and social care goals.

57 Seyfang, G (2002) *The Time of Our Lives*, Central Books.

58 Extract from the London Time Bank, www.timebanks.co.uk.

Printed in the UK for The Stationery Office Limited
on behalf of the Controller of Her Majesty's Stationery Office
177788 03/05